52
·WAYS·TO·
PREVENT
HEART
DISEASE

52
·WAYS·TO·
PREVENT
HEART
DISEASE

Terry T. Shintani, M.D., M.P.H.
and
J. M. T. Miller

OLIVER
NELSON

THOMAS NELSON PUBLISHERS
Nashville

Published in Nashville, Tennessee, by Oliver-Nelson Books, a division of Thomas Nelson, Inc., Publishers, and distributed in Canada by Word Communications, Ltd., Richmond, British Columbia.

Printed in the United States of America.

Library of Congress Cataloging-in-Publication Data

Shintani, Terry T., 1951–
    52 ways to prevent heart disease / Terry T. Shintani and J.M.T. Miller.
        p.   cm.
    Includes bibliographical references.
    ISBN 0-8407-9671-4 (pbk.)
    1. Coronary heart disease—Prevention. I. Miller, J. M. T. (Janice M. T.), 1944– . II. Title. III. Title: Fifty-two ways to prevent heart disease.
RC685.C6S517   1993
616.1'2305—dc20   93-4089
                                                                        CIP

        1 2 3 4 5 6 — 98 97 96 95 94 93

CONTENTS

THE EXERCISE CONNECTION

THE SOCIAL CONNECTION

1

UNDERSTAND THE PROBLEM

Nine Jumbo Jets Let's put heart disease into perspective by comparing it to another cause of death. Currently, airline tragedies strike somewhere in the world every other week or so. You see the headlines.

And every time one of these tragedies occurs, the entire nation is instantly abuzz: How can we prevent these needless deaths? It's a legitimate concern. But what if *every single day of the year* a 747 crashed—and that crash might have been prevented? Can you imagine the public outcry?

And yet every single day, heart and vascular disease kills the equivalent of the passenger load on not just one but *nine* jumbo jets crashing every single day of the year, not just this year but next year and the next and the year thereafter. And on and on this continues and will continue until we at last come to our senses and implement the many things we can do to prevent this tragedy known as heart disease.

America's Number One Killer   According to *The U.S. Surgeon General's Report on Nutrition and Health,* odds that you'll die from cardiovascular disease are well over 43 percent.[1] Cardiovascular disease kills nearly as many Americans as all other diseases *combined.* In fact, just one aspect of cardiovascular disease—coronary heart disease—is currently responsible for one-fourth of all American deaths.

The Personal and Financial Costs   In 1989, an estimated 944,688 Americans died because of cardiovascular disease (CVD). That's one death every thirty-two seconds. And death is only part of the tragedy. About 1.5 million people suffer and/or die from heart attacks each year. Nearly 500,000 more have CVD-related strokes. And then there are the countless hours of misery spent in surgery, in painful recovery, in disability, in a family's grief, and in worry about how to pay the bills. CVD's financial cost to our economy and our health system in 1992 alone was a staggering $108.9 billion.

To get a feeling for the scope of the problem, look around you. Statistically, one in every four people you see already has CVD, and almost half of all the people you know or meet will die from this disease.

The Good News   On the brighter side, we now know that most CVD is preventable and/or treatable; that includes the most common form of CVD, coronary heart disease/atherosclerosis, the disease that will be the focus of this book.

We can at last see the way toward a final and complete solution. Indeed, we have already made more headway against coronary heart disease than against any of the other major degenerative diseases.

In the 1950s and 1960s, the death rate from coronary heart disease (CHD) reached a peak. That was about the time researchers began to understand some of the more salient aspects of the disease. In the past decade, the changes implemented through resultant discoveries are being reflected in the statistics. The rates of CHD have fallen over 25 percent, and they continue to fall as more and more people learn the truth about the causes and preventive measures. Despite the decrease, however, heart disease is by far the number one killer of all Americans.

Stop the Epidemic!   We *can* stop this epidemic in its tracks. And we can begin right now, today. Researchers are teaching us that all we have to do is to change our life-styles and nutrition, and within a few years we could reduce the number of people who die from heart and other cardiovascular disease from nearly a million a year to a fraction of that. There's already been a decrease over the past two decades, so we know we can make a difference. It's possible. But it's going to take some work.

What Can You Do?   You can lower the odds that you or someone you love will fall victim to this modern-day plague by changing your diet and life-style. That may seem like an overwhelming task but don't despair. Just read on, and you'll learn what you need to do to keep the plague from your and your family's door.

About This Book This book is designed so you can assimilate and incorporate one new preventive measure each and every week of the year. If you follow the advice you learn here, you'll be doing your part to find the total solution to this most devastating of all diseases. Your part of the solution can begin right now with your heart and circulatory system. At this very minute, biochemical forces at work in your body are determining whether or not you will be one of the unfortunates or one of the "lucky" ones. Believe it or not, you have complete control over most of those forces, no matter how old you are, no matter how poor or good your health.

We can stop almost all coronary heart disease. The question is, will we?

Will *you?*

THE
INFORMATION
CONNECTION

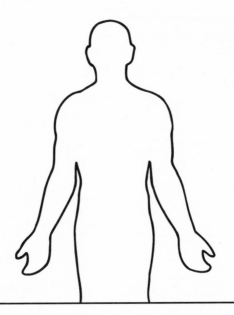

2

UNDERSTAND
YOUR
HEART

Get Acquainted   You carry inside you one of the greatest wonders of the world. It is a machine that pumps ceaselessly, daily moving 4,300 gallons of blood over an approximate distance of 216,000 miles 365 days a year. It has an electrical system that fires an impulse without fail about 38 million times per year to stimulate the heartbeat, and it does this year after year, rain or shine, light or dark without resting. It doesn't heat up or create any noise or pollution. Its engineer must be preeminent to have created such a marvel. What is this wondrous creation?

Just inside your left breast lies a hollow muscular organ about the size of your fist—your heart. If you press the flat of your hand to that area, you'll feel a rhythmic pulsating, or thumping. That's your heartbeat. Your heart beats because certain nerve impulses stimulate certain muscle fibers, causing them to contract, then expand, contract, then expand, to pump your blood to every cell, tissue, and organ of your entire body, providing oxygen, nourishment, and life.

Your heart has to be strong to do this job. It will pump twenty-four hours a day, seven days a week, throughout the entirety of your physical existence. It will push blood through miles and miles of conduits known as arteries, vessels, and capillaries, while it also carries waste products and carbon dioxide back to the lungs or other areas where they can be expelled.

Your Cardiovascular System   The word *cardiovascular* is composed of two Greek words: *cardio* (*kardia,* meaning "heart") and *vascular* (derived from the Latin *vasculum,* which means "vessel"). It denotes the entire system of the human heart and all the blood vessels, arteries, and capillaries that it supplies.[1] The heart is so intricately involved with the workings of the blood that most people think of it all as one single system. This system is also known as the *circulatory system,* and the two terms are used interchangeably.

Now you know what we mean when we talk about cardiovascular disease. It is, basically, any disease that has to do with the heart/blood system. In the next section, you'll learn the various types of heart disease. There are many, and they have various causes and treatments. But the type of disease that this book will primarily talk about is atherosclerosis, the most common type of heart disease. In fact, it is currently responsible for one-fourth of all American deaths. And we now know what to do to prevent almost all of it. So, why are so many people dying?

Let's look again at the scope of the problem. Nearly

four thousand Americans will have heart attacks today. Nearly one-third of them will be fatal. Some forty million people in this country have diagnosed cardiovascular disease. Many more people have this disease but don't yet realize it. Are you, or will you be, one of these people? The answer to that depends on many factors and on what you choose to do about them. You've already made the first step toward escaping this catastrophe just by reading this book. If you incorporate the advice you'll find here into your life-style, you'll be well on your way to beating the odds for good!

3

UNDERSTAND HEART DISEASE

The Number One Killer Of the approximately 759,400 Americans who die yearly from heart disease, some 500,000 die from atherosclerotic heart disease. That makes atherosclerotic heart disease the number one killer in America. When most of us say "heart disease," we usually mean atherosclerotic heart disease. But there are other forms of heart disease.

Other Heart Disease *Congenital heart disease* includes diseases that people may be born with, such as congenital valve problems in which the valve does not develop normally. It is a frequent cause of heart murmurs.

Infectious heart disease includes viral infections and bacterial infections. Viral infections usually affect the heart muscle, and bacterial infections usually infect the valve and cause valvular problems such as bacterial endocarditis.

Rheumatic heart disease is a collection of heart problems caused by inflammation, which follows infection by a specific strain of streptococcus called beta-hemolytic Group A streptococcus.

Hypertensive heart disease is caused by the heart's having to work very hard due to the high pressure in the blood system. Usually, the heart becomes thickened as a result of overwork and eventually goes into congestive heart failure.

Other forms of heart disease include cardiomyopathy, alcoholic heart disease, and tumors to name a few.

Back to the Number One Killer   For the purposes of this book, as we said earlier, we are dealing almost exclusively with atherosclerotic heart disease. Atherosclerosis results from the narrowing or blockage of arteries that feed the heart and supply it with blood, oxygen, and nutrients. The main cause of this disease is the buildup of cholesterol plaque on the inside of the coronary arteries.

The buildup of cholesterol plaque takes place over many years, and the narrowing is very gradual. Thus, there are usually no symptoms until the arteries are almost completely blocked. When the arteries become very narrow as a result of the buildup, blood supply to the heart is impaired, and sufferers will likely experience chest pain.

When a physician determines that the chest pain is a result of a narrowing of the arteries, the chest pain is called *angina pectoris.* This pain may occur intermittently; the contraction of blood vessels may contribute to the feeling of chest pain when the contractions cause the already narrowed arteries to nearly or completely close for short periods of time.

Often, the edges of cholesterol plaque will be rough, and small clots may form at these rough edges. Usually, these clots will disappear naturally through the body's normal mechanism. However, if the artery is narrowed a great deal, even a small clot can completely block the flow of blood through that artery. When such a complete blockage occurs, a heart attack results. The purpose of this book is to teach you 52 things that can keep that from happening.

4

KNOW THAT IT'S NEVER TOO LATE

Feeling Too Old to Change?   Conventional wisdom tells us that as we get older, our hearts just wear out. There's no point in trying to fight back. And it is true that the risk of heart disease increases with age. But does it have to?

The answer to that is yes and no. Yes, your body does eventually wear out, and that includes your heart. But no, you do not have to sit back and wait as your heart inevitably gives out long before the rest of your body. The current epidemic of heart disease is more a factor of life-style and diet than of physiological inevitability. You *can* actively and successfully pursue a healthy heart, all the days of your life.

It was once thought that atherosclerosis was irreversible and something you had to live with once you got it. Treatment was and often still is relegated to the use of medications to cover up the signs and symptoms of atherosclerosis. Keep the blood pressure low, relax the heart and blood vessels, thin the blood, and if all that didn't work, resort to surgery to bypass the problem. All the while, it was known that in animal experiments atherosclerosis could be reversed with a healthy diet. It was also known that a decrease in cholesterol caused an almost immediate decrease in the risk of heart attack. Further studies showed that medication and/or diet alone could achieve this effect.

For years in my private practice, I've treated chest pains and heart disease with a good diet, and I've had excellent results. Then, in 1990 a study was published indicating that a low-fat diet could not only prevent heart disease but literally reverse it. The patient who showed the most improvement in study was a man of seventy-four who had had severe coronary blockage for many years before starting the program. Other people in the same age bracket had similar results.[1]

Down and Out in Norway   During World War II in Norway, dietary fat and cholesterol intake was forced down to a minimum as people had to give up their typical high-fat, meat-centered diets because of rationing and reduction in the food supply. Surprisingly, the rate of heart disease went down almost immediately and in an almost identical statistical curve to the reduction in intake of fats. And it didn't matter how old the person was. Reductions in heart disease rates were found in people between the ages of forty and sixty, sixty and eighty, and even over eighty years old.[2] The effect of changing your diet on heart disease is both rapid and impervious to age.

5

KNOW YOUR RISK FACTORS

Avoidable Risk Factors   The primary avoid-able risks for heart disease are these:

- High blood (serum) cholesterol
- Bad diet
- Smoking
- Obesity
- Lack of exercise
- Other diseases such as diabetes and hypertension

Let's look at them one at a time.

High serum cholesterol   It is so closely related to heart disease that for every 1 percent increase in cho-lesterol in your blood, there is a 2 percent increase in risk of heart attack. The reverse is also true. If you lower your blood cholesterol by 1 percent, you'll lower your risk of heart attack by 2 percent.[1]

Bad diet   In countries where people eat a lot of fat and cholesterol, heart disease rates are significantly higher than in other countries. The evidence is clear. Eating a high-fat, high-cholesterol diet increases your risk of heart disease.

Smoking   Smoking is known to cause cancer, but many people are unaware that smoking also causes heart disease. Death from heart disease in smokers is significantly higher than in nonsmokers.

Obesity   Excess body weight correlates with higher risk of heart attack. Of the main types of obesity, apple-shaped obesity, that is, increase in fat around the belly and upper body, more commonly found in men, seems to be a greater risk factor for heart disease than does the pear-shaped obesity seen in most obese women.

Lack of exercise   Sedentary people have poorly conditioned hearts; therefore, when a heart attack does occur, they are far less likely to survive. But exercise plays an even more crucial role in the prevention of heart disease. It tends to improve the good cholesterol versus total cholesterol ratio. However, exercise alone isn't enough. A good diet is an equally vital factor in preventing heart disease.

Other diseases   The most common diseases other than high cholesterol that contribute to atherosclerotic heart disease are diabetes and hypertension. We'll talk about them at length later, but for the moment you need to know that they are included as preventable risk factors because both diseases *can* be prevented through life-style and diet, as can most heart disease. If you have these diseases, keep them under control; you'll be winning the battle against the devastation they can directly cause to your body, and you'll also be doing all you can to prevent the risk of heart attack.

Unavoidable Risk Factors Some risk factors cannot be avoided. Nevertheless, you should know about them. If you are at high risk, you can heighten your vigilance, then do all that's necessary to change your life-style and more diligently practice the 52 ways to prevent heart disease. These risk factors include the following:

• Family history
• Being male
• Being a postmenopausal woman
• Age

Family history If any blood relatives have had a heart attack or have had a history of high cholesterol or high blood pressure, you should be even more vigilant than most people. Heart disease tends to run in families, and the closer the blood relative, the greater your risk. You *must* do something to decrease your risk.

Being male For some reason, female hormones tend to protect women against heart disease. Men tend to die at a much higher rate than do women.

Being a postmenopausal woman However, after menopause women's risk of heart disease tends to catch up with that of men. That seems to be due to diminishing hormone production. Hormone replace-

17

ment therapy may be one way to combat this deficiency. However, this therapy brings with it risks of its own. So before you use hormones, be sure to consult your physician.

Age As you get older, the risk of heart attack tends to increase. You'll be happy to know, however, that in many countries it is not a significant problem. If you change your diet and life-style to preventive ones, you have a better chance of avoiding heart disease, no matter what your age or location. In the famous Framingham Heart Study, not one single person with a cholesterol level lower than 150 died of a heart attack, and the results were the same for all age groups, young or old.

Now you know your risk factors for heart disease, both avoidable and unavoidable. It's time to determine which ones apply to you and what you can do to protect yourself. Read the next section and immediately put it to use.

6

CHANGE YOUR DIET—NOW!

Stop Eating the SAD   Despite much quibbling over specifics, even the most pessimistic doctors and researchers agree that there is a lot wrong with the Standard American Diet (which has the appropriate acronym SAD). In fact, the most important risk factor for heart disease—serum cholesterol—is determined primarily by the food you eat. So to prevent heart disease, you have to change your diet and change it now!

The Framingham Study   We'll be talking a lot about cholesterol in this book because of the direct relationship between cholesterol and heart disease. In one of the largest CHD studies ever done, the Framingham Study (so-called because it took place in Framingham, Massachusetts), twenty thousand men were evaluated for over forty years, and of those people, no one with cholesterol levels of 150 or less died of a heart attack. That was regardless of stress level, age, level of exercise, smoking, family history, or other diseases present, including hypertension. The study also showed that there was, indeed, a direct correlation between heart disease and cholesterol.[1]

Back to Norway We've already mentioned what happened to the people in Norway during the war. In the accidental study, as dietary fat intake decreased dramatically from 1940 to 1945, the death rate from heart disease decreased—beginning almost immediately. What we didn't tell you was that *after* the war, when the dietary fat intake returned to its prewar levels, death rates from heart disease leaped back up to the high prewar level.[2]

Cut Your Risk Now This and other studies offer strong evidence that changing to a low-fat, low-cholesterol diet can make a rapid and long-term difference in whether or not you suffer or die from a heart attack. So follow the dietary advice offered in "The Nutrition Connection." Don't dig your grave with your fork and teeth. Change your diet, and you may save your life!

7

PROTECT YOUR CHILDREN AGAINST HEART DISEASE

Recognize the Culprits Many of us have heart disease today because our parents unwittingly failed to protect us against it.

Not that we can blame our parents. Until recently, most people had no idea about what caused heart disease. The idea that diet and life-style were primary culprits had the medical establishment arguing for years, so how could our parents have known?

Kids and Cholesterol But now we do know that heart disease starts early in life. Although there are really no outward signs and symptoms of the problem, pediatric surgeons have noted finding cholesterol-caused atherosclerotic plaque in very young children. Parents make food choices for young children. Thus, if you're not careful, you may well be setting the stage for your children's future heart attacks.

The rules for prevention of heart disease are the same for children as for adults except that it is important to make sure that children on a very low-fat diet get adequate calories and nutrients. Most Americans are raised on and live their whole lives ingesting diets loaded with cholesterol and fats. We pass this way of eating down to our children. That's how we set the stage for their future heart attacks.

In addition to fostering a bad diet, some of us pass on the nasty habit of smoking, which our children learn by imitation. They also learn not to exercise; instead, they watch TV and are otherwise inactive. Many of us pass along genetic predispositions toward heart disease to our children. Much as we regret this, nobody can change heredity. But whether or not the genetic predisposition toward the disease that you pass on is a strong one, you can provide an environment that helps your children adopt a life-style that will likely prevent heart disease, not trigger it.

8

LEARN
HOW TO
PROTECT YOUR
CHILDREN

What Can You Do? Here are a few things you can do to give your children the best possible chance of beating the odds against heart disease. It's entirely possible that our generation could be the last one that has to battle heart disease as an epidemic! Wouldn't that be wonderful?

1. Don't feed your children high-cholesterol foods This book offers a number of dietary tips. It's very important that you try to incorporate this advice into your family's meals, not just your own. Heart disease usually takes many years to develop, and the time to start preventing it is during childhood. The trick in getting your children to eat right is to provide tasty, healthy alternatives to the junk food and fast foods they eat today. Make sure that healthy snacks are available, for example, fruits, oil-free popcorn, and rice cakes. Whole grain cereals make excellent snacks.

2. Stop smoking   There is a direct link between smoking and heart disease. That smoke you breathe out and your children breathe in can cause them all kinds of health problems. And if you smoke, you also give your children the impression that it's okay for them to smoke. You may be fostering a lifelong habit that is deadly not only to your children but to your grandchildren.

3. Cut the fat   In any case, stop feeding your children fried foods, and that includes fast foods, which are mostly fried. Discover the alternatives. Kids love fresh fruit and air-popped popcorn. Favorites such as pizza, burritos, tacos, pasta, and baked potatoes provide the whole family with a nice break from meat-centered meals. These foods can be made low-fat by easing up on or eliminating cheese, oil, and butter and eliminating meat. They're also far easier on the pocketbook, as are almost all superhealthy foods.

4. Give your children life-style options   Provide healthy choices, such as low-fat, no-cholesterol foods, alcohol-free and smoke-free environments, and opportunities for exercise. Then let them decide. With smaller children, you'll have an easier task.

5. Be a good example   All children will learn by your example, and the best thing you can do to keep from giving your children heart disease is to change your life-style and diet and let them know why!

9

MAINTAIN
AN IDEAL
WEIGHT

Live Long and Prosper   Mortality from heart disease correlates to body weight, which means that those of us who are overweight are much more likely to die young from a heart attack.

A large percentage of overweight people die from heart attacks. Indeed, almost all of the controllable heart disease risk factors go up with obesity: the risk of diabetes increases; cholesterol increases; the risk of high blood pressure increases. Therefore, you can combat heart disease by attaining and then maintaining your ideal weight.

The Fat Gram Approach   One of the best ways to lose weight is to eat a diet that is very low in fat. Limiting the grams of fat you eat appears to be a generally healthy and reasonable way to lose weight. In this approach, you would limit your fat intake to no more than 10 to 15 percent of your calories. For a

person who eats 2,000 calories (the caloric requirement for a medium-sized moderately active woman
in her thirties), this means no more than 22 grams of
fat per day. If you want to go for an initial reduction
to 15 percent fat, you can eat no more than 33 grams
of fat per day.

Body weight apparently decreases in direct correlation to your consumption of dietary fat. This seems
to hold true regardless of how much you eat, so if you
just watch the percentages, you can forget counting
calories.

Bring on the Bulk   But you also have to consider the bulk in the foods you eat. If you're consuming mostly sugar or candy that contains no fat at all
(such as jelly beans), you can gain weight because
these foods are highly concentrated in calories.

Bulk is essential to a viable human diet. If you
aren't getting adequate dietary bulk, you'll feel dis-
satisfied and continue eating till the craving for bulk
is satiated. So, the best way to lose weight is to eat
low-fat foods that are bulky and fill up the stomach,
such as brown rice, broccoli, carrots, and potatoes.

Give Up Your Yo-Yo   Many people are con-
stantly gaining weight, then losing it, then gaining it
back, and so on. Called yo-yo dieting, this is a dangerous approach to weight control. A study in the October 21, 1992, issue of the *Journal of the American
Medical Association* concludes, "Both body weight
loss and weight gain are associated with significantly
increased mortality from all causes and from coronary heart disease but not from cancer."[1] In other
words, give your heart a gift: achieve your ideal
weight gradually and sensibly, and then stay there.

10

LEARN THE TRUTH ABOUT ASPIRIN

An Old Drug with Some New Tricks? Aspirin has been around for nearly a century, but only recently have researchers begun to suspect that it might have an effect in the prevention of heart disease. One researcher, Dr. Charles H. Hennekens of the Harvard Medical School, directed a double-blind study that made the headlines.

In the double-blind study, certain physicians were given aspirin while others were given placebos. In 1987, the first hard data were processed and showed that the aspirin group had developed 44 percent fewer cases of heart disease than had the placebo takers.[1]

So pleased was the research team by these results that "the monitoring board decided to terminate the aspirin study and to share its findings quickly—and possibly save millions from experiencing heart attack."[2]

Caveat Emptor Still, aspirin is far from a miracle drug. As promising as these results may be, it won't do you a bit of good to sit down and inhale a lard-laden prime rib, then pop a few after-dinner aspirins as an antidote.

Nevertheless, in appropriate circumstances, aspirin may be useful. In some cases, aspirin prevents heart attacks and strokes. It does this by thinning the blood and thereby minimizing the risk of clotting. Many factors must be taken into consideration, however, when someone is taking aspirin on the regular basis necessary to fight heart disease. Aspirin can increase the risk of bleeding, which is why your surgeon will always tell you not to take any aspirin for a certain time before surgery. Before taking aspirin, you should consult your physician so all the variables can be discussed and added into the decision of what dosage and type of aspirin—if any—will best keep you healthy in all capacities, including your heart.

11

GET REGULAR MEDICAL CHECKUPS

What About Symptoms?   One of the most dangerous aspects of heart disease is that in the early stages there are no symptoms. Heart disease usually takes decades to develop. But if risk factors are detected early, you can attack the problems that can lead to heart disease before they attack you.

These dangerous risk factors do not show symptoms in their early stages:

• High cholesterol
• High blood pressure
• Diabetes mellitus

Because they are silent risk factors, you need to get regular medical checkups so that you'll know whether or not you have any of these problems or even tendencies toward these problems.

The AHA Says   The American Heart Association (AHA) recommends a physical exam every five
years, starting at age twenty, including screening for
these risk factors. The association emphasizes that
older people may need checkups more often. People
with a history of heart disease or with additional risk
factors may require more frequent medical examina-
tions. Some physicians recommend a physical exam
every two years after age forty, and every year after
age fifty.

Ask your doctor about screening tests for cholesterol and diabetes. We'll talk more about diabetes in
a separate section, but you need to know that like
early stage heart disease, this one can be a killer.
And it's doubly so, since it can contribute to heart
disease. Make sure you get your blood pressure
checked regularly. It's one place where trouble can
show up well in advance of any serious problems and
in plenty of time to prevent them.

Give Up Fear   Most of all, don't be afraid of
what you'll learn. Even if you find out that you have
potential or early stage problems, regular checkups
can enable you to detect them in ample time to do
something about them and protect yourself against
having a heart attack.

12

UNDERSTAND YOUR BLOOD PRESSURE

What Is Blood Pressure?   Blood pressure is the force with which your blood is moved through your bloodstream. It is determined in part by the beating of the heart and thus moves in pulses through your blood system. Other elements that determine blood pressure are the resistance in the blood vessels (how narrow they are) and, to a lesser extent, the amount of fluid in your bloodstream.

What Is Normal Blood Pressure?   We all know now that high blood pressure is a risk factor for heart disease. Keeping it normal will reduce the risk of having a heart attack. But most of us don't know what "normal" is.

From your doctor's point of view, normal blood pressure is approximately 120 over 80, give or take 20 points for the systolic, the higher number, and 10 points for the diastolic, the lower number. However, in younger and thinner people, blood pressure may be normal at slightly below this range.

What Are They Measuring?   Just what does all this mean? It's really pretty simple when you take it apart and look at it.

Systolic   The systolic represents the highest pressure in your blood system when your heart is beating and pulsing the blood through your bloodstream. You feel the ebb and flow of this pressure when you take the pulse on your wrist or on the carotid artery in your neck. Normal for this is around 120, and abnormally high is over 140.

Diastolic   The diastolic, which is the lower number, represents the lowest pressure in the arteries of your blood system, that is, the pressure in the ebb between heartbeats or pulses. Normal for this is about 80; high is over 90.

Putting it all together   Ideally, both numbers should be within the normal range. But it is most important to keep the lower number (diastolic) in the ideal range. This is because a high diastolic pressure is more of a risk factor than a high systolic pressure.

What Causes High Blood Pressure?   High blood pressure can be caused by a number of factors.

Narrowing or clogging of the arteries   By far the most common cause of high blood pressure is narrowing of the arteries due to atherosclerosis, or too much cholesterol. As we've already pointed out, when plaque builds up inside your arteries, it forces the blood to travel at higher pressure, just like when you put your thumb on a hose when watering a lawn.

A heart that pumps too hard   It may be the result of a hormonal imbalance or stress, or one of a number of other causes.

Too much salt in the diet   Only about 40 percent of people with high blood pressure are salt sensitive, so this isn't a problem for everyone. But for those who are sensitive, it can be risky.

Kidney problems   Changes in the pressure regulatory mechanisms can occur as a result of kidney disease, and they can also be caused by a host of other ills. The kidneys play an important role in helping regulate blood pressure.

13

LEARN TO CONTROL YOUR BLOOD PRESSURE

How to Get Control of Your Blood Pressure

Now you know what blood pressure is. But what can you do about it if it's giving you trouble?

Check with your doctor   First of all, you should check with your doctor about this vital aspect of your health. Except in unusual circumstances, each person has the capability of determining blood pressure. Actually, several key things can easily make the difference. We'll list them for you below, then talk about each one in more detail in other sections of this book:

- Change your diet.
- Lose some weight.
- Exercise correctly (which probably means exercise more).
- If your doctor prescribes medication, take it faithfully.

Watch your diet   By the way, if your blood pressure exceeds 140 over 90, *always* see your physician, who may or may not recommend medications. Whatever is advised, be sure that you also try the dietary approach. Even if your blood pressure is controlled with medication, your risk for heart attack remains unless you lower your cholesterol to around 150.[1]

High blood pressure can mean latent cardiovascular disease. Always take abnormal blood pressure seriously, and take the appropriate steps to keep yours normal.

14

KNOW THE
DIABETES
CONNECTION

A Serious Risk Factor   As you've seen, diabetes is a serious risk factor for heart disease. Heart disease is more common among people with diabetes, it has an earlier onset, and it is usually more severe.

What Is Diabetes?   Diabetes is the body's inability to handle blood sugar. In the human body, insulin is required to move sugar from the bloodstream into the body's cells, where it can be used as energy. Adult onset (Type II) diabetes is a disease in which insulin somehow doesn't work as well as it should. It is often correlated with a high-fat diet and obesity. In adult onset diabetes, the disease can usually be controlled through diet, exercise, and other medication. Insulin may be added as a medication in severe cases. However, if persons with adult onset diabetes miss an insulin dose, the consequences are usually not severe. Because of this, adult onset diabetes is also known as non–insulin-dependent diabetes mellitus, or NIDDM.

On the other hand, with juvenile onset diabetes (Type I), insulin is absolutely required. In this disease, the cells in the pancreas (where insulin is produced) have been destroyed by an autoimmune phenomenon: that is, the body attacks its own cells. Thus, people with juvenile onset diabetes produce no insulin rather than have ineffective insulin, as in adult onset diabetes. This disease usually begins at a very young age and hence its nickname of juvenile onset diabetes. If these individuals do not take insulin as prescribed, they may develop diabetic keto-acidosis and may risk death. This type of diabetes is also known as insulin-dependent diabetes mellitus (IDDM).

It is vital that you know whether or not you have either disease because you must keep your blood sugar under control. That, as you have seen, is one reason you need to get regular medical checkups. And after you've seen your doctor, if you discover you have any form of diabetes, follow your physician's instructions carefully. They will usually include recommendations for diet and exercise patterns and perhaps also dosages of medication.

The Heart Connection   Scientists are not sure why, but the high levels of sugar in the blood seem to cause abnormality in the ways in which fats and cholesterol are handled. Apparently, the result is an acceleration of the depositing of plaque in the arteries, which increases your risk of heart attack. So ask your physician about screening for diabetes, and know the diabetes connection.

15

KNOW THE HORMONAL LINK

The Unavoidable Risk You will recall that being a postmenopausal woman is one of the unavoidable risk factors for heart disease. After menopause, a woman's risk of heart disease tends to catch up with that of a man. That seems to be due to diminishing production of female hormones. We don't yet understand the complexities of hormonal balance and how it relates to heart disease, but studies indicate that hormones tend to have a protective effect.

Hormone replacement therapy is one way to combat the postmenopausal risk, but most physicians carefully weigh the risks against the benefits when they're considering this therapy.

Estrogen Estrogen apparently works on the cholesterol levels in the bloodstream, and helps give women a better cholesterol risk profile than men. Unfortunately, estrogen replacement is also correlated with an increased risk of uterine endometrial and breast cancers. In fact, tamoxifen, a drug used to treat breast cancer, is actually an estrogen blocker.

This added risk of cancer can apparently be minimized by combining the estrogen with progesterone, a male hormonal replacement. But this combination decreases the efficacy of the prevention against heart disease.

What to Do?   The question of hormonal replacement is a complex one, and postmenopausal women should definitely talk to their physicians and discuss every aspect of the pros and cons before considering hormonal replacement therapy as a preventive measure against heart disease. As is true with the use of any medication, the potential benefits must be weighed against the risks. Numerous aspects of personal health and health history will apply. This decision should be made on a completely individual basis in consultation with a physician.

16

LEARN
YOUR
WARNING
SIGNALS

Early Warnings Save Lives   Learn the early warning signs and symptoms of heart disease. If an impending heart attack is detected early, much can be done with modern technology to improve your odds of surviving even a severe attack. Today, everything from bypass surgery to angioplasty to anticlotting therapy to simple things like aspirin can be used in an emergency situation by the physician to prevent sudden death from heart attack.

But how do you know if you're having a heart attack? You should know about several general symptoms.

Know Your Symptoms   A typical heart attack is manifested by left-sided chest pain or tightness or heaviness or discomfort. Sometimes it is accompanied by a radiation of pain to your back, your jaw, or your left shoulder or arm. Sometimes it is accompanied by shortness of breath, increased perspiration, and a feeling of fatigue. If any of these symptoms come on suddenly or become chronic, check with your doctor immediately.

Heart attacks can also manifest themselves in an atypical manner. You may get a feeling of persistent indigestion accompanied by one or more of the other signals. Or a heart attack may come on with a sensation of someone sitting on your chest but no real chest pain. At other times, it may be an unexplained tingling of the jaw or of the left arm or shoulder. And sometimes people have silent heart attacks; there are no or few symptoms, or the symptom is a feeling of tiredness or lack of stamina.

Because of the many ways in which heart disease can manifest itself, you should be aware of the major and unmistakable symptoms and also the vague, seemingly benign symptoms that can give you an early warning. Know all these signals. And if you have any one of them, contact your doctor immediately. Symptoms may occur early enough to help save your life but then disappear, even though you're still in danger.

A Fortuitous Flight   On a plane flying to Boston, the flight attendant paged any doctor on board. I responded and found a gentleman experiencing tightness in his chest. After evaluating the patient, I immediately asked the pilot to have an ambulance waiting upon landing. I then gave the patient one of the few medications we had on board, nitroglycerine, under the tongue to see if the chest pain would disappear. After a second pill, the symptoms resolved themselves at just about the time the plane landed. The patient felt good again. He did not want to go in the ambulance. He argued that he had things to do and would see his own doctor the next day.

I insisted that he go directly to the emergency room, by ambulance, as quickly as possible. I felt that he might be having a heart attack that was still in progress. I warned him of the possibility of sudden death. He finally agreed, though reluctantly, and left the airport in the ambulance. Two days later, the patient's son phoned to tell me, "You saved my father's life." He went on to explain that his father had indeed been having a heart attack but reached the emergency room in time for them to implement anticlotting therapy and minimize damage to his heart.

Such an event points out that the signs and symptoms of heart attack may or may not be evident, especially to the patient. But usually, you'll have some indication (though possibly small) that something is wrong. At that point, contact a physician immediately. It may save your life.

THE
TOBACCO
CONNECTION

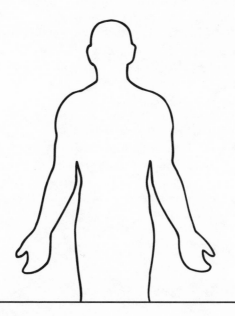

17

DON'T
SMOKE

The Chronic Killer Most people know that smoking contributes to cancer, the second leading killer of Americans. But most people don't realize that it also contributes to heart disease, the leading killer. Warnings by the U.S. Surgeon General have appeared on every cigarette package in the United States for years. Yet, our government does not prohibit the sale of cigarettes, even though taxes from tobacco sales don't offset the $70 billion spent annually in health-care costs for smoking-related illnesses.

In fact, since smoking contributes to both heart disease and cancer, estimates are that smoking contributes to one in five of all the deaths in this country! One study of 119,404 female nurses showed that smoking "was associated with a twofold to threefold increase in the risk of fatal coronary heart disease or nonfatal infarction. Overall, cigarette smoking accounted for approximately half these events."[1]

The American Heart Association tells us that

> people who smoke a pack of cigarettes a day have more than twice the risk of heart attack of people who have never smoked. And people who smoke two or more packs have a risk of heart attack three times greater. Smokers who have a heart attack have less chance of surviving than nonsmokers. And smokers who continue to smoke after having a heart attack increase the chances that they'll have a second attack.[2]

Deadly When Used as Directed Cigarettes are the only major American product allowed on the open market that can lead to death when used as directed. One police officer who had been stricken with lung cancer made the point in some anticancer commercials that the cigarettes in his pocket were far more dangerous than the bullets in his gun. And he was right because more people die each year from smoking-related illnesses than are killed by all the handguns in this country.

How the Killer Works Smokers have more atherosclerosis than nonsmokers. Perhaps that is because smoking can result in increased heart rate and blood pressure, forcing the heart to work harder and requiring more oxygen, while at the same time carbon monoxide from smoking decreases oxygen-carrying capacity. Smoking can lower the levels of high-density lipoprotein, or HDL, which is good cholesterol. Cigarette smoking also seems to increase clotting and, therefore, makes it more likely that a heart attack may occur in a narrowed vessel.

18

DON'T FORCE YOUR KIDS TO SMOKE

Passive Smoking   Maybe all that information in 17, "Don't Smoke," doesn't matter to you. If it doesn't, consider this: in 1986, the U.S. Surgeon General and the National Academy of Sciences reached the conclusion that smoking causes health problems in those who are breathing smoke-polluted air. The Surgeon General's report asserted for the first time that segregating smokers into separate areas in the same room does nothing at all to help the passive victims of cigarette smoke.[1]

Furthermore, numerous studies examining the effects of parental smoking on respiratory illness in their children demonstrate an increased incidence of both upper and lower respiratory problems among young children of smoking parents as compared with children of nonsmoking parents.[2] Similar studies show correlations between smoking parents and increased risk of certain infectious and other diseases.

It was as if when parents smoked, the children were smoking, too.

Think About It   Even if you don't care what you do to yourself, think of the others who have no control over the smoke you exhale into the air: your friends, your family, and your children. One of the best things you can do to protect yourself—and them —against heart disease is to *stop smoking and stop right now!* Then you won't be forcing your kids to smoke.

19

UNDERSTAND YOUR ADDICTION

For Addicts Only   If you're already addicted to nicotine, you know that it isn't easy to quit smoking. Some experts say it's just as difficult or even more difficult to break an addiction to tobacco as it is to break one to heroin or alcohol. The dynamics are the same. You have a physical addiction as well as a habituation, which means that the behavior of smoking tobacco is so integrated into your daily behavior that quitting means overhauling your entire behavioral patterning.

Withdrawal   Nicotine will almost completely disappear from your system within one day after you completely stop smoking. In withdrawal you may experience headaches and serious irritability, among other unpleasant effects. But physical withdrawal is just a matter of realizing that your body is ridding itself of poisons and is chemically realigning itself to exist without them. It will pass. The hard part is changing your smoking-centered behavior. Many people who'd like to quit can't make it past that hurdle.

Break Your Addiction There are several ways to stop smoking. Some people quit cold turkey. They suddenly realize how expensive their habits are, in terms of finances and health, see red, and stop. Others need help. Fortunately, these days plenty of help can be found. Most legitimate self-help groups work if you're serious. Or you can see your physician. Some doctors prescribe nicotine gum to replace cigarettes. It gradually decreases the nicotine input into your body and minimizes the actual withdrawal symptoms. Others have started prescribing the nicotine patch, which adheres to the skin and does much the same thing. Whatever way you choose, you can make it past the initial nicotine withdrawal.

Break Your Habituation The hard part is going to be the first few months as you literally rearrange your life. Until you begin doing this, you'll never realize just how much a smoker's life revolves around tobacco.

The most important factor of beating your addiction is to understand exactly what you're going through so that when those gnawing nudges of discontent attack you at certain times of the day, you'll see them for what they are. Once you consciously recognize them, you can take control over them.

20

REPLACE A BAD HABIT WITH A GOOD ONE

When Did You Smoke? Most smokers are habituated to having a cigarette (or other nicotine product) at certain times of day: after a meal or before bed, for example. To begin to understand just how firmly tobacco used to control your behavior, you need to sit down and make a list of when you used to smoke. They are going to be your problem times. Next, you need to make a list of behaviors that you can use at those times to replace the behavior of smoking.

You're giving up a negative behavior. Replace it with something positive. One person who had the early stages of emphysema fought off urges to have a cigarette by replacing the smoking behavior with deep breathing exercises. "I used to tell myself that I had to do fifty long, slow, deep breaths," she said, "and then if I still wanted a cigarette, I could have one."

The strategy worked for her in two ways: (1) it gave her a behavior with which to replace the activity of shaking a cigarette out of the package, lighting it, and inhaling, and (2) the deep breathing brought more oxygen into her bloodstream, thereby relaxing her. It also brought her addictive-habituated behavior to the forefront of her consciousness and allowed her to fight back.

Things to Do   You could choose from many positive things to supplant smoking behavior. A few of them are listed here:

- Get physical exercise. Even a few simple stretches might make the difference.
- Chew gum.
- Have a snack. Make sure it's a healthy one, or you'll trade one problem for another.
- Do deep breathing exercises.
- Start a penny jar. Calculate the cost of each cigarette you used to smoke, then drop the pennies into the jar each time you want a cigarette. Earmark the money for something really special. And by the way, if you sit down and calculate the money you spend in a year on cigarettes, you're guaranteed to be amazed. (Most estimations run upward of $1,000 for an average habit.)

You could also pick out a few of your favorite things to do as a reward for your ongoing commitment to stop smoking. In time, your new, healthy habits will become natural. Then you'll wonder why you waited so long to stop smoking.

21

JOIN
THE
BATTLE

What Battle?   The American Medical Association (AMA) has vowed to work toward a smoke-free society by the year 2000. Now that you've seen what smoking does to you and your loved ones, and now that you don't smoke (if you ever did), you can help to discourage others from starting.

A Toxic Cloud Over the Tobacco Industry?
The winds of change are blowing in a healthy direction. A recent Supreme Court ruling gives ill smokers the right to seek damages against cigarette companies; it "allows those who suffer health effects from smoking to sue tobacco companies for allegedly misrepresenting the dangers of their products" and is " 'another nail in the coffin of the tobacco industry,' said Lonnie Bristow, M.D., of the AMA's board of trustees. He said it may lead the American public to 'rise up and attack cigarette advertising.' "[1]

In Australia,

> Ms. Liesel Scholem, a 65-year-old psychologist, has won £35,000 after a two and a half week court case found that her health has suffered from passive smoking. Ms. Scholem, backed by the Non-Smokers' Movement of Australia, sued her former employer, the New South Wales Health Department, alleging that between 1974 and 1986, when she worked as a counsellor for mental health patients at a community health center, she had been exposed to tobacco smoke. . . . Almost half the staff and the patients at the center had smoked, and there was no air conditioning.[2]

Things are starting to change.

Protecting the Children   The AMA is also after Joe Camel, the subversive symbol that encourages all cartoon-loving people—kids included—to smoke his brand. The AMA's July 1992 rally against smoking "was led by U.S. Surgeon General Antonia Novello, M.D., and focused on the impact the ads have had on the nation's children. According to Dr. Bristow, in the three years since Joe Camel ads have appeared, the ratio of smoking teens whose brand is Camels has risen to 30% from 3%."[3]

Tobacco companies also sponsor sports events, giving the impression that they actually encourage good health; they send people on speaking tours to tout the First Amendment rights that (they say) guarantee them the right to continue marketing their pollutants to the world (and never mind our rights to the facts about our health and to clean lungs and air).

Start today. Write a letter to the editor. Write to your legislators. Talk about it with your friends. You can help to win this fight against heart disease.

THE
CHOLESTEROL
CONNECTION

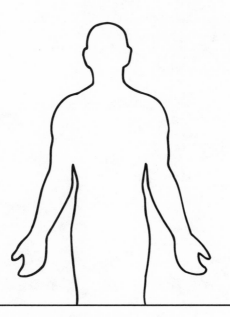

22

GET
YOUR
CHOLESTEROL
TESTED

Coming to Terms with the Killer   A direct relationship between diet and heart disease, and especially between the "bad" cholesterol and atherosclerosis, is very clear. In fact, in the late 1980s the National Cholesterol Education Program (NCEP) issued an emphatic recommendation that all adults get their cholesterol tested in an effort to at last come to terms with the number one killer.

The Basics   It's so easy to get tested that no one has any excuse not to know the cholesterol count.
  You can get tested in one of two ways:

- The simple way is to get it done through a Department of Health or a cholesterol screening program, which is often held at a shopping mall or another public setting. They use the finger-stick method; a drop of blood is taken and put in a machine, which can give you the results within three minutes. You can call your Department of Health to find out if it has free or low-cost programs of this kind.

- However, the simple tests aren't as accurate as those done at a laboratory on blood taken by needle from one of your veins. Your physician can arrange this test, which is much more accurate because the lab uses more sophisticated machines to test the blood. The results take a day or two, but when you get them, you know a more precise cholesterol count. Insurance may or may not cover the cost, so you need to be aware that this testing may be a more expensive choice.

Guidelines   If you want to prevent heart disease, the best thing you can do is to keep your cholesterol low. For every 1 percent increase in your cholesterol, there is a 2 percent increase in your risk of having a heart attack.

The national guidelines indicate that the desirable cholesterol level is below 200 mg/dl. An ideal level is around 150 to 160 mg/dl, based on the Framingham Heart Study.[1] Cholesterol levels between 200 and 240 are considered to be a moderate risk, and those 240 and above are definitely high risk. Estimates are that over 50 percent of all Americans have cholesterol in the undesirable (over 200) level.

If you're in that category, you need to take charge of your health. So get tested, whether you take the simple test or the more precise one. If you take the simple one and you find your cholesterol is over 200, see your physician to discuss getting the more precise one done. Cholesterol is your best indicator of the health of your heart. So get your cholesterol tested. You could save your life.

23

KNOW YOUR CHOLESTEROL

The Good, the Bad, and the Deadly It is well established that heart disease is directly related to total blood cholesterol. But there is another way to get an even better view of your risks of getting heart disease: by knowing the type of cholesterol in your body.

There are two main types of cholesterol, and only one of them is dangerous. But before we introduce these two types, let's take a general look at cholesterol and what it does.

What's in a Name? The French scientist Chevreul named cholesterol after the Greek words *chole,* meaning "bile," and *sterol,* meaning "solid." It is a vital part of every human or animal body. It helps build cell membranes; it creates bile acids, forms the nucleus of vitamin D and sex hormones, and is otherwise essential to life.

However, you don't have to eat cholesterol to get your supply. Your body makes quite enough in your liver. But many foods contain cholesterol, and that is where you get into trouble. Today's diets reek with excess cholesterol. When too much cholesterol finds its way into the bloodstream, the balance is dangerously tilted. Fats in your diet, especially saturated fats, contribute to the problem.

Cholesterol is waxy in texture, and the blood can't dissolve it. It begins to accumulate inside the arterial walls, building up and narrowing the artery, thus setting the stage for heart disease. Cholesterol is carried in the bloodstream in clusters of molecules known as *lipoproteins*. There are two basic types: good and bad (deadly).

If you know you have high cholesterol, it's a good idea to talk to your physician and get your cholesterol level fractionated in a special blood test so that you can tell how much good cholesterol you have compared to the bad.

Good Cholesterol   "Good" cholesterol is also known as HDL cholesterol, or high-density lipoprotein cholesterol. They are called high-density lipoproteins because they contain little fat and cholesterol; therefore, they are high in density and don't easily float. The particles of HDL cholesterol tend to carry the plaque out of your arteries and carry it to the liver to be processed. An easy way to differentiate between the good and the bad is to remember that *H* equates with *healthy*.

Bad Cholesterol   The "bad" cholesterol is known as LDL cholesterol, or low-density lipoprotein cholesterol. One way to remember this is to know that oil floats, which means it is low in density.

LDL is bad for you because it is laden with oils, fats, and cholesterol (all of which are low in density), and it delivers all this into the artery walls.

Guidelines If your total cholesterol level is higher than about 160, HDL is actually a better predictor of heart disease than your total cholesterol count. In other words, the higher the HDL, the lower the risk of heart disease. And conversely, the lower the HDL, the higher the risk of heart disease. In general, in men an HDL below 45 is considered too low. In women, below 55 is considered too low. (These values may vary slightly from lab to lab.) The significance of your HDL level depends on how high or low your cholesterol is. If your cholesterol is below 150, a low HDL doesn't mean much. If your cholesterol is over 200 and your HDL is below 35, you are at high risk.

Because there is an interaction between HDL and total cholesterol in assessing your risk, most labs will report the ratio between your total cholesterol and your HDL, so you know not only how much cholesterol you have but how much of it is good and how much is potentially deadly. The lower the ratio of HDL to total cholesterol, the lower your risk of heart disease. The higher the number, the higher your risk. An average ratio of cholesterol over HDL for women is about 4.44, and an average ratio for men is about 4.97. Remember that men and women with average ratios are at risk, so it is important to have a ratio lower than average.

24

LEARN TO CONTROL YOUR CHOLESTEROL

What Can You Do? Because of the strong, direct relationship between a high cholesterol count and heart disease, it is crucial that you keep your cholesterol within the approved guidelines. The first step was to learn your cholesterol count. But now that you've had your test and you know it's too high, what can you do about it?

The first thing, of course, is to cut down on your dietary intake of cholesterol. In the next section, you'll learn a rule to help you find cholesterol and learn how to avoid it.

The second thing is to give up most dietary fats. In "The Nutrition Connection," you'll learn in detail all you need to know about fat to stay healthy. You'll learn how to limit your intake of fried foods, fatty animal foods, oils, ice cream, and other high-cholesterol, high-fat food.

The third thing you can do is to cut down on saturated fats. Saturated fats tend to raise cholesterol more than other types of fat.

The fourth thing that will improve your cholesterol rating is to exercise regularly. It will do more to raise your HDL (your good cholesterol) than lower your total cholesterol. You will find several suggestions about exercise in "The Exercise Connection."

Finally, you need to look carefully at other parts of your life-style. Smoking is a contributor to high cholesterol. Studies suggest that drinking too much coffee may elevate your cholesterol levels.

Heed Nutrition Facts Most of all, follow the nutrition guidelines in this book. If "people perish for lack of understanding," don't let yourself remain unschooled about the substances you put into your body. Make no mistake about it: what you eat or don't eat can cost you your life.

25

LEARN TO FIND CHOLESTEROL IN YOUR DIET

Where Is It? You certainly know by now that dietary cholesterol is bad for you. But how do you translate this knowledge into practical, applicable advice?

You can use one simple rule to identify the dietary sources of cholesterol: *anything with a face on it contains cholesterol.*

Conspicuous Cholesterol That's right, animals, fish, chicken, poultry, shrimp, crabs, lobsters—all have faces, and all have cholesterol. That includes dairy products and eggs, which come from cattle and poultry—which both have faces. Things like grains, vegetables, fruits, and beans have no faces and, therefore, no cholesterol. This is one reason vegetarians tend to have less heart disease than do people who eat animal flesh.

THE NUTRITION CONNECTION

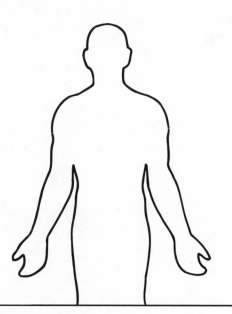

26

KNOW YOUR NUTRITION

Healthy Foods Mean Healthy Bodies You are what you eat. That's trite but true. If we eat healthy foods, we'll have healthy bodies. If we eat unhealthy foods, we'll have poor health. So true is this fact that according to current statistics, approximately 70 percent of us are dying of diet-related diseases. In a nutshell, most of us are ignoring our nutrition.

The topics related to nutrition are going to help you rectify that, while they also give you direct information that will help you and your loved ones prevent heart disease. And you're going to learn some fascinating things about yourself and your body in the process.

Food for Thought   Did you know that

- eating five or more servings of vegetables and/or fruits a day can go a long way toward keeping you healthy?
- many of the degenerative diseases that are killing us are related to the amount of fat in our diet?
- there's a lot more fat to red meat than meets the eye?
- substituting poultry for red meat may be a major mistake?
- Eskimos may know something about heart disease that you don't?
- dairy products are, in general, bad for your heart?

You're about to learn all this and more. So read on to learn just what you need to know to keep a heart attack from *your* door.

27

LEARN
FIVE
FOR YOUR
HEART

Five Fitness Rules   In October 1991, the National Institutes of Health (NIH) kicked off a campaign to help Americans learn to eat right. Their advice is short and sweet:

1. Eat five servings of fruits and vegetables a day.
2. Eat at least one vitamin A–rich selection every day.
3. Eat at least one vitamin C–rich selection every day.
4. Eat at least one high-fiber selection every day.
5. Eat cabbage family (cruciferous) vegetables several times each week.

They define *one serving* as "½ cup of fruit, ¾ cup of juice, ½ cup cooked vegetable, 1 cup leafy vegetable, or ¼ cup dried fruit."[1] Doesn't sound too hard, does it?

Eat Your Five, Stay Alive! Why is this important? First of all, vegetables and fruits have no cholesterol in them. They are also high in fiber and low in fat content. These qualities help to lower cholesterol. And fruits and vegetables are chock-full of other nutrients that keep you generally healthy.

So eat your five or more servings of fruits and vegetables per day, as well as your other food. They're sure to help you prevent heart disease.

28

CUT
THE
FAT

High Fat and Heart Attacks   We have
learned that fat intake contributes to heart disease.
Epidemiological studies, which compare the heart
disease rates from country to country, show a direct
correlation: the greater the fat intake, the greater
the heart disease rate. Clinical studies back up this
correlation. There is also ample evidence that excessive and incorrect use of dietary fats contributes to
premature aging, many types of cancer, diabetes, and
many other human problems, including most fatal
heart disease.

The AHA Recommends   The American Heart
Association has been a leader in the hue and cry
against dietary fat. Currently, it recommends that
dietary fat intake be less than 30 percent of your total
calories. Most Americans now consume somewhere
between 37 and 40 percent of their calories as fat.
   Evidence suggests that even lower levels of fat in-

take would lead to lower rates of heart disease. Recently, the diet of Chinese people was compared to that of Americans of Chinese ancestry living in the United States. The researchers discovered that the level of fat intake in the diet of the Chinese living in China was about half that of their American counterparts and their heart disease rate was very low. Americans of Chinese ancestry, on the other hand, had heart disease rates similar to those of other Americans.[1] These studies clearly show that the differences are not genetic and are more likely due to differences in diet.

Other studies show direct correlations between amounts of dietary fat and the amount of cholesterol in the blood.

How Much Fat?   In 1989, my colleagues and I conducted a study that determined that a diet as low as 7 to 12 percent in fat would lower cholesterol levels and even lower blood fat (triglyceride) levels, which is another risk factor for heart disease. The 7 to 12 percent fat diet is also high in complex carbohydrates and fiber, which lowered the blood pressure in persons with high blood pressure. We hypothesized that such a diet could not only lower risk factors but might also reverse atherosclerosis.[2]

In 1990, Dr. Dean Ornish published his landmark study showing that a similar diet with about 10 percent of calories from fat could not only prevent heart disease but reverse it. Patients with radiographically demonstrated atherosclerosis reversed their arterial narrowing by eating a 10 percent fat diet. The arteries that were narrowed due to cholesterol started to open up, and the chest pain and other symptoms of heart disease slowly disappeared.[3]

29

KNOW
YOUR
FATS

The Most Deadly Fat   Even though we generally need to cut the fat in our diets, the most deadly
fat, and therefore the one we *most* need to be aware
of, is saturated fat.

Types of Fat   But what is saturated fat? To understand it, we need to learn the types of dietary fat
and how to distinguish one from another.

Saturated fat   This fat is found in fatty substances
that are solid at room temperature. Saturated fat is
most often found in lard and butter and other animal
fats, as well as in tropical oils, such as coconut and
palm oil. The saturated fats are worse than polyunsaturates and monounsaturates because they tend to
raise cholesterol more than the others.

Polyunsaturated fat   Fatty substances containing this fat tend to be liquid at room temperature. The common sources of this fat are most vegetable oils, including the highly popular corn oil that makes up most of our cooking oils.

Monounsaturated fat   Fatty substances containing this fat also tend to be liquid at room temperature. This type of fat is easiest on your heart—on your body in general, for that matter. You can find it in olive oil and canola oil. Of all the various oils, these tend to raise cholesterol the least.

However, we can't always say to ourselves, "Well, this fat is solid at room temperature; therefore, it's saturated, and I should be careful not to eat it." Or "It's liquid and therefore okay." The whole thing is a bit more complicated than that.

The confusion arises because of the ways in which our foods are processed. Technologists at food companies often change polyunsaturated and monounsaturated fats so they will be solid at room temperature. They do this through the process of hydrogenation. And in this process, hydrogenated vegetable oils become saturated fats. If you're eating processed food, sometimes all bets are off. In the process of processing foods, the original chemical composition can often become so bent and twisted and contorted that the original food almost ceases to exist. This is true not only of oils and fats but of all foods. Try to eat your foods as lightly processed as possible. Fresh fruits, nuts, vegetables, whole grains—these are always your best dietary bets, whether you're taking care of your heart or just your general health.

And your best strategy is to decrease *all* the fats

and oils in your diet. General governmental dietary guidelines suggest that 10 percent of our calories come from saturated fats, 10 percent from polyunsaturates, and 10 percent from monounsaturates. But general dietary guidelines are invariably conservative and designed as recommendations for the general public rather than as an ideal for a motivated individual. In truth, the best policy is to keep all your fat and oil intake low.

Dr. Ornish's study demonstrated that the 30 percent formula currently recommended by the AHA actually caused a *progression* in heart disease. Our work in Hawaii used only 7 percent of calories from fat and demonstrated a 14 percent reduction in cholesterol. These findings suggest that people can do just fine on very low-fat diets, and most of them are healthier than ever before.

In particular, watch out for saturated fat. Ease up on animal foods, tropical oils, and hydrogenated vegetable oils, and you'll be doing a lot to protect yourself against this epidemic of heart disease.

30

LEARN THE FAT FINDER'S FORMULA

The Truth About Food Labeling   It's essential that you learn how to identify the fats in your diet if you're going to lower your risk of getting heart disease and other degenerative diseases. Yet how can you do that when the fat information on food labels contains some of the most subtle deceptions in modern marketing? The fats in foods are often hidden or skillfully disguised on the food labels—and deliberately so. This may be one reason for this epidemic of heart disease.

Did You Know?   Are you aware that

- light, low-cal mayonnaise contains 90 percent fat?
- 91 percent fat-free burgers are about 50 percent fat by calories?
- hot dogs are about 83 percent fat? (They should be called fat dogs.)

These examples make it obvious that you can't always believe what you read on food labels. You might think that 2 percent fat milk is good because it is only 2 percent in fat. But 2 percent fat milk is 2 percent fat by weight, not by calories. However, most of our health recommendations regarding fat are expressed as a percentage of calories. If you look at 2 percent milk by calories, it is actually about 35 percent fat! In fact, whole milk is only 3.3 percent fat by weight but is 55 percent fat by calories. And so on.

You now know that the ideal anti–heart disease diet is approximately 10 to 15 percent fat by calories, as based on recent studies. But it's going to be impossible for you to reach this ideal without knowing how much fat is in the food you purchase, prepare, and eat.

Become a "Fat" Detective   If you're going to beat the bad nutrition you've been addicted to and protect your heart, you have to learn how to be a "fat" detective. You have to be on the alert for fat fraud during every supermarket trip, every dinner party, every food-centered outing.

How do you become a "fat" detective? This is where the Fat Finder's Formula comes in. The Fat Finder's Formula (FFF) is like Sherlock Holmes's magnifying glass. It offers you a way to look right past the apparent nutritional contents of any given product and see to the "heart" of things.

Fighting Back with the FFF   Here's the formula. Take the grams of fat (usually found on the food label now), and multiply them by 9 (the number of fat calories per gram), then divide the answer by the total number of calories in the food. Your answer will give you the proportion of fat as a decimal figure. To convert this to a percentage, simply multiply by 100.

A good example is hot dogs, which are supposedly less than 30 percent fat. In reality, when the hot dog is 30 percent fat by weight, it turns out to be 83 percent fat by calories! And it is the percentage of fat per calories that matters, and that physicians talk about when they tell you to cut back your fat intake to 35 percent or 20 percent or even 10 percent. Chicken hot dogs (which are often labeled as being less than 20 percent fat) are not much better. Using the FFF, you realize that chicken hot dogs are about 73 percent fat.

Work to Stop Deceptive Food Labeling

Since it's apparent now that too much dietary fat has severe consequences for the American public health, it's long past time that these deceptive practices were stopped. In 1993 or 1994, laws will be enacted to tighten control over deceptive practices. It remains to be seen how well the laws will be implemented. The task is a formidable one, and the federal government is snowed under with the work it is already doing in that regard. For the moment, you're on your own to detect the fat in your food. Fortunately, the FFF gives you a way to calculate the deception and get to the truth.[1]

31

EASE UP ON THE RED MEAT

Stop Eating Seared Flesh   A friend of mine surprised a group of us at a cookout by asking, "Are you eating the seared flesh of dead animals?" He was trying to make the point that red meat is bad for your health.

The statement evoked a disgusting image that stayed with me. I hope it will stay with you because it makes a good point.

What Goes Around Comes Around?   It is a strange justice that as human beings kill millions of animals, the animals ultimately wind up killing millions of us! When we eat so much animal food, we are our own worst enemies.

Heart disease, as we've said so often, is the number one killer of all Americans. And heart disease is directly related to the amount of cholesterol and saturated fat that we eat. Animal food is high in these deadly nutrients, for example:

- A 3.5 ounce portion of beef contains about 91 mg of cholesterol, which is very high.
- If we eat organ meats, that is, foods such as livers and intestines, the cholesterol levels are even higher. For example, a 4 ounce piece of liver has 410 mg of cholesterol.

Higher Grade Equals Better?   The United States Department of Agriculture (USDA) grades meats by their fat content, or marbling. The higher the fat content, the higher the grade. This rating gives a false impression that a high grade meat is high quality. Nothing could be more untrue: the higher the grade, the worse it is for your heart and your overall health because of the higher fat content.

Meats, in general, are very high in fat content. Consider these amounts by calories:

- A slice of beef is 71 percent fat.
- A hamburger patty is 63 percent fat.
- A lean hamburger patty is 59 percent fat.
- And 91 percent fat-free burgers are, when measured by percentage of calories, about 50 percent fat. Furthermore, the fat is mostly saturated, the type that is most likely to clog your blood vessels.

In short, if you want to prevent heart disease, follow some friendly advice: ease up on eating the seared flesh of dead animals.

32

EASE UP ON THE POULTRY

Chicken or Beef? A lot of people are talking about how good chicken is for you. You may have already decided to switch from beef or pork to chicken. Sorry to say, that's not such a good idea.

- A 3.5 ounce portion of chicken has about 85 mg of cholesterol.
- A 3.5 ounce portion of beef has about 91 mg of cholesterol.

Not much difference, is there?

But why, then, are so many people, including physicians, recommending that we eat less red meat and more chicken? I can only presume the recommendations are made because the fat content of chicken, when compared with that of beef or pork, looks healthier. And it is true that when you *do* eat chicken, you can remove the skin and reduce the total fat and the saturated fat content of the food, thus gaining some advantage.

Beyond Fat   The problem is, only a few people seem to be looking beyond overall fat content to the health impact of the cholesterol content of poultry. I like to ask my students, "How much do you lower the percentage of cholesterol in chicken when you remove the skin?" I always surprise them with the answer: "None. Because cholesterol is in every cell of all animals, including fish and fowl, the percentage stays the same—with or without skin. Therefore, the lean part of the chicken still contains approximately the same percentage of cholesterol as does the fatty part."

- A 3 ounce fried chicken breast is 47 percent fat with 89 mg cholesterol.
- A 3 ounce skinless roasted breast is 21 percent fat with 84 mg cholesterol.

Nothing Gained   As if that weren't enough, many of us further complicate the problem by eating chicken fried in other fats. Even if you are disciplined enough to remove the skin before you eat fried chicken, you're kidding yourself if you think that really helps. During the frying process, the fat melts and seeps into the meaty part of the chicken, and you end up consuming a great deal of fat even if you have removed the skin.

So switching from beef and pork to chicken is just trading one problem for another. The fact is, switching from red meat to poultry provides no substantial reduction in cholesterol and possibly but not necessarily a reduction of fat levels in the diet.

33

KNOW YOUR
FISH
AND
FISH OILS

Learning from the Eskimos   In 1972, an important study determined that Greenland Eskimos who ate a relatively high-fat, high-cholesterol diet had much less heart disease than did Eskimos who lived in Denmark and ate a similarly high-fat, high-cholesterol diet but with a content that was similar to the regular European diet.[1] This finding stimulated a lot of research because it seemed to contradict the widely held notion that high fat meant high heart disease.

In the 1980s, much of the research focused on fish oils because the indication was that something the indigenous Greenland Eskimos were eating was protecting them from heart disease. The substance, whatever it was, was suspected to be found in the fish, sea mammals, and wild game that made up their primary diet.

The Omega-3s   Subsequent research showed that the fish of the Arctic Eskimos contained a certain type of oil not found, or found in very small quantities, in other forms of animal food. These oils are known as Omega-3 fatty acids.

Omega-3 fatty acids caused three notable effects that helped prevent heart disease.

1. They thinned the blood, that is, made it more difficult for clots to occur   As we described in chapter 3, two things need to happen for a heart attack to occur. First, there must be a narrowing of the arteries, usually through cholesterol deposits (plaque) in the arteries. Second, a little clot must form on the rough edges of the atherosclerotic plaque to plug the narrowed opening of the blood vessel. By thinning the blood, the Omega-3s kept the blood from clotting and blocking the artery. The heart attack was prevented. The downside was that it was possible for blood to be thinned too much, and Eskimos died of hemorrhagic strokes (that is, bleeding strokes) at a much higher rate than their European counterparts.

2. Increased consumption of Omega-3 fatty acids caused a significant decrease in blood fats and triglycerides   Triglycerides are a co–risk factor for heart disease.

3. There was a slight decrease in cholesterol levels

Eat Your Fish?   So we know that Omega-3 fatty acids can have a preventive effect on heart disease. Some proponents use this as justification for promoting the use of fish oil pills. However, we must be cautious about recommending pills when the research has been done on a whole food.

A better way to prevent heart disease is to avoid cholesterol altogether. No matter how good the Omega-3s may be, fish has a face. Which means it contains a significant amount of cholesterol, which means that at the same time you're ingesting those Omega-3s, you're ingesting cholesterol.

Still, contemporary experts continue to tell us that eating fish is a good bet—especially cold-water fatty fish—because they are rich in the Omega-3 fatty acids. And a lot of doctors are telling their patients to give up eating so much red meat and poultry and substitute fish. A study in the May 9, 1985, issue of the *New England Journal of Medicine,* concluded, "The consumption of as little as 1 or 2 fish dishes per week may be of preventive value in relation to coronary heart disease."[2] The researchers reached this conclusion after they established that the consumption of fish apparently reduces heart disease. This finding suggests that if you're going to eat fish oils, it's better to get them from fish than from a capsule on the shelf of your health food store.

Do or Don't Eat Fish   Other studies suggest that it's even better to avoid cholesterol-containing foods altogether. A study of vegetarians in the Boston area indicated that their average cholesterol was 125, which suggests that their heart disease risk was nearly zero. The vegetarians' average cholesterol rating was a whole lot better than the rating for those people who ate fish and other cholesterol-containing foods as well.

34

EASE UP
ON THE
DAIRY
PRODUCTS

Calcium and Cows   Calcium is important to the human body, and for years we've been told that the best source of calcium is dairy food. To be sure, dairy food contains calcium. But most dairy food also contains cholesterol and saturated fat.

The U.S. Surgeon General's Report on Nutrition and Health recommends that we keep our serum cholesterol below 200 mg/dl and our cholesterol intake below 300 mg per day. It's difficult to achieve this standard if you're eating much dairy food. For example, consider that

- whole milk has 32 mg of cholesterol per cup.
- 2 percent milk has 18 mg of cholesterol per cup.
- cheddar cheese has about 105 mg of cholesterol per 3.5 ounce portion.
- American cheese has 94.5 mg of cholesterol per 3.5 ounce portion.

Fats   Furthermore, the fat content in dairy food is generally high. In whole milk, it is 55 percent. As we've seen, 2 percent milk is especially misleading because it is actually 35 percent fat by calories. One percent milk isn't much better. It is actually 25 percent fat by calorie (remember, this is what the experts are talking about when they talk about fat content percentages and optimal diets).

As for the fat in cheese, cheddar cheese is actually 74 percent fat by calorie, and most other types of cheese are similarly high in fat, although some new ones are lower.

Skim Milk?   From the perspective of heart disease, perhaps the only acceptable form of dairy food is skim milk products. Skim milk is so named because the fat is skimmed off; therefore, it has almost no cholesterol or fat. However, skim milk does have potential problems associated with it.

Other Problems with Milk   Dairy food is a major source of allergy and is associated with diseases such as asthma and juvenile onset diabetes.[1] In addition, 70 percent of the world is lactose intolerant, that is, sensitive to lactose, a milk sugar found in all dairy products.

Substitutes   Better sources of calcium include broccoli, leafy greens such as kale and collard greens, and seaweeds. They are low in fat and contain no cholesterol. And if you're really worried about calcium intake, you can turn to calcium supplements.

35

EASE UP ON THE EGGS

The Eggs and I   Eggs are a source of high quality protein. Unfortunately, they also have one of the highest cholesterol contents of any food.

One egg contains 213 mg of cholesterol, all of it in the yolk. By comparison, one 3 ounce slice of roast beef contains about 73 mg of cholesterol. In other words, one egg contains almost as much cholesterol as three moderate portions of roast beef!

The egg is also 62 percent fat by calories. And like the cholesterol, all of the fat is in the yolk.

It's No Yolk   If you must eat an egg, take out the yolk. What's left is egg white, otherwise known as egg albumin. It's almost pure protein. However, as good as egg protein is, we are now finding that most Americans eat way too much protein, especially animal protein. This excess can cause a loss of calcium in the urine, which may promote osteoporosis.

36

FIND A
HEALTHY
SOURCE OF
PROTEIN

Creating the Protein Myth   Protein has definitely been overpromoted in the past few decades. The need for protein has long been the main justification for the high consumption of meats, poultry, and even dairy food in our society. Unfortunately, decades ago, when the emphasis on protein began, the researchers had no idea that they were promoting foods that would one day be shown to contribute to heart disease, cancer, and most of the other killer diseases that plague America today.

Furthermore, we have recently learned that we don't need as much protein as we once thought. We have also found that instead of eating too little protein, Americans are eating too much.

Killing the Protein Myth Before It Kills Us
Most of the people I see in my practice are eating 200 to 400 percent as much protein as they need. And

even in my vegetarian patients, I have yet to see a protein deficiency. The old belief about vegetable proteins being "incomplete" proteins is not true. Just about all grains, beans, and vegetables, when prepared and eaten in their whole form, have adequate protein. Some amino acids may be lower in some of these foods than in others. But if you calculate the amino acid content in these whole foods, you'll find that if you eat enough of them to meet your daily requirement of calories, your intake of amino acids will be adequate.[1]

So even people eating a whole food vegetarian diet get adequate amounts of protein if they're not eating empty calories in the form of fats and sugars. Furthermore, they get ample protein without taking in all the fats and toxins that accompany it in meat, poultry, fish, and dairy products. Remember, fats are highly implicated in heart disease.

So get your protein from beans, grains, and vegetables. Ease up on the meat. Diets high in animal protein correlate with shortened life spans in industrialized populations. The protein myth is dead. Eat enough whole grains, vegetables, and beans and you'll certainly get enough protein.

37

KNOW YOUR NIACIN

Vitamin B$_3$ Niacin is also known as vitamin B$_3$. Another name for it is nicotinic acid (as opposed to nicotinamide). It stands head and shoulders over the other vitamins as a cholesterol fighter. And though diet is still the main choice, the National Cholesterol Education Program has listed niacin as a primary choice in cholesterol control. It works directly on the liver and helps to raise your levels of good cholesterol.

Niacin is available in most health food stores. But don't rush right out and buy a bottle. Some people can't take niacin. Their reactions are too severe. And even for those people who can take it, a word of caution is warranted. Though niacin is a water-soluble vitamin and it is generally quite safe to take in supplemental form so long as you stay within the guidelines of the Recommended Daily Allowance (RDA), the dosage required to begin lowering your cholesterol is substantially larger than the RDA. At these pharmacologic dosages, side effects can range from mild to severe.

See Your M.D.   *Never* take large dosages of niacin without being supervised by your doctor. The therapeutic range for this vitamin is from 1 to 3 grams (1000 to 3000 mg), and some physicians prescribe even more. The possible side effects at these dosages include heavy flushing, shortness of breath, stomach upset, headaches, ulcers, and other possible problems. Your doctor will want to know about any of them and will regulate your dosage accordingly.

Niacin in large doses can damage your liver. Your liver manufactures cholesterol, and niacin works by interfering with this manufacturing process. Your liver is vital to your overall health, so it is even more important that you have medical supervision if you're taking the large dosages of niacin required for cholesterol control. Your doctor will want to do liver function tests and keep track of what's happening. Still, niacin is an effective cholesterol fighter and may have fewer side effects than other medication used to fight cholesterol. It may be a good choice. However, don't forget that changing your diet is still the best approach to fighting cholesterol. If you want to try niacin as a cholesterol fighter, see your M.D. first.

38

EAT
PLENTY
OF FIBER

The Fiber Factor Many countries have far
fewer cases of heart disease than does the United
States, and people in those countries also eat more
fiber, according to authority Dr. Dennis Burkitt.[1]
They eat more whole, unprocessed grains, beans, and
fresh vegetables and fruits—just the sort of diet we
need. Modern medical science seems to be pointing
us more and more toward the old natural styles of
eating.

High-fiber diets help prevent heart disease. In the
1980s, studies concluded that oat bran eaten once a
day is effective in lowering cholesterol. The substance in oat bran presumed to lower cholesterol is
the soluble fiber. Other research quickly showed that
while oat bran is an excellent source of soluble fiber,
other sources, such as whole grain, would also lower
cholesterol.

The Two Types   Fiber is the nondigestable part of grains, vegetables, and fruits. There are two types, soluble and insoluble.

Soluble fiber   This includes pectins and gums, which are found in certain legumes, fruits, vegetables, and whole grains. These substances appear to bind the cholesterol in the gut and carry it out of the body, reducing the amount absorbed and thus helping to lower overall cholesterol.

Insoluble fiber   This is so called because it does not dissolve in water. This type of fiber increases your stool bulk and helps it pass quickly and smoothly through your intestinal tract. Though there is no clear correlation between this type of fiber and lowered risk of heart disease, ample evidence indicates that insoluble fiber contributes to your overall good health and may help to prevent colon cancer and other intestinal diseases.

Most foods of plant origin contain plenty of both types of fiber, so long as they aren't refined.

Psyllium Husks   Fiber is so effective in lowering cholesterol that the husks from psyllium are commonly used in medical practices to help patients lower their cholesterol. The beauty of using this substance is that it is natural, is never absorbed into the bloodstream, and has few, if any, side effects. A word of caution, however. If you have gastrointestinal problems, consult your physician before adding psyllium husks to your diet.

Fiber-Rich Foods   Any number of health-enhancing foods contain high amounts of both types of fiber. We've heard from advertisers that oat bran is best. But almost all whole grains, whole vegetables, and whole fruits are excellent sources of fiber. We can get ample amounts of fiber from cruciferous vegetables (broccoli, cauliflower, cabbage, brussels sprouts, turnips, spinach, and rutabagas), other vegetables (carrots, celery, asparagus, etc.), fruits (blackberries, apples, peaches, raisins, etc.) as well as beans, seeds, and all types of whole grains.

Fiber-rich foods include some of the tastiest foods around. So if you want to lower your risk of heart disease and at the same time improve your overall health, these are the foods for you.

39

EAT
WHOLE
GRAINS

The Germ of the Wheat During the days of ancient China and Egypt (most likely), someone decided that rice and breads could be improved upon by separating the germ from the bran. The first bowl of white rice and the first slice of white bread were born. Both became symbols of status in various parts of the world, whereas the coarser whole grain breads and brown rice were eaten by the "unfortunate."

In our prosperous country, white bread and white rice have long since ceased to be status symbols. Today, we think of them as staples. This is unfortunate because we now know that these foods are less healthy than whole foods.

White vs. Whole In the 1980s, after the fiber studies had won over the hearts of medical scientists, studies showed that whole grains possessed similar cholesterol-controlling abilities. They contain a significant amount of both soluble and insoluble fiber. But when you mill, or refine, grains, you strip away most of their cholesterol-fighting ability.

Whole Foods   It's time to make the point that God created our foods to fit our bodies. All the nutritional components of any whole food are made to perfectly complement each other and to interact with perfect symmetry to nourish our bodies. Take away any one component, and you've ruined the balance that is the basis for perfect health. For example, our bodies need B complex to digest starches. We should marvel at the fact that there is ample B complex in the bran of the whole grain. Mill the bran off the grain and you remove the B complex. Excessive consumption of white rice only can actually result in beriberi.

Other Benefits   And speaking of perfect health, an additional advantage of eating whole grains is that they provide a good source of calories that are low in fat and are low in cholesterol. Healthy servings of whole grains replace foods that might otherwise be high fat and harmful. For example,

• brown rice is only 7 percent fat.
• whole wheat flour is only 5 percent fat.
• whole wheat bread is only 12 percent fat.
• corn is only 9 percent fat.
• oats are only 15 percent fat.

And none of these contain any cholesterol.

Finally, you should start eating whole grains because they just plain taste good.

40

BE
A SMART
SHOPPER

Your Goal   The place to begin preventing heart disease is in the supermarket. Don't kid yourself that the half-gallon of rich ice cream is going to sit in your freezer while you eat only half a bowl a month or that it's just for the kids. (Why would you do that to them anyway?) Learning to shop wisely is the first step toward attaining a healthy life-style.

To recap some of what you've learned, while shopping, you'll want to:

- avoid or limit cholesterol-containing foods, which include animal, poultry, and fish food and their products, such as eggs and cheese.
- remember that animal food also contains a lot of saturated fat, which is bad for your heart.
- choose a lot of whole grain products.
- select enough fruits and vegetables to eat five servings a day.

Purchase Some Implements   As your budget permits, purchase kitchen implements that will help you prepare healthy foods. A vegetable steamer will be helpful in preparing your vegetables and other tasty dishes. You can purchase a stainless steel one for well under $20 anywhere in the United States. Or you can purchase one of the newer model steamer/ rice cookers. Black & Decker has an excellent one for around $40. It simplifies the process of cooking vegetables to the point that it may well make the difference in whether or not you eat your veggies.

A food processor is excellent for making your own baby foods and has a thousand other uses. The cost is $50 and up.

A grater will be useful for slicing vegetables and otherwise preparing food. If you don't already own one, buy one made of stainless steel for well under $10.

A food blender is great for making shakes, smoothies, soups, and hundreds of other foods. You'll spend somewhere in the neighborhood of $50 to $250 for a good one.

A pressure cooker will simplify cooking whole grains. It will cost about $75–$100.

Buying Your Food   Stock up on an ample supply of whole grains. You might also want to buy a recipe book teaching you how to make delicious whole grain dishes. Make them, instead of meats, the center of your new, healthier diet.

Fresh produce is especially important. You should eat as much as you want. If at all possible, buy organic vegetables and fruits. If you can't, don't be overly concerned. The cholesterol in all animal foods and the fats in many foods are far more dangerous than the pesticides that you might find on some produce. A quick bath in soap and water will get rid of most of the pesticides anyway.

Select a variety of foods. Be adventuresome; try foods that you have never tried before. And don't be discouraged. No matter where you live, you'll be surprised at the variety of vegetables available to you once you step beyond the conventional potatoes, tomatoes, corn, and beans that you grew up with. Stay away from canned vegetables as much as possible, by the way. The best is fresh, then frozen. Use canned only as a last resort unless you're ambitious enough to do your own canning so you can control quality and ingredients.

The advice given above with regard to vegetables is also true for fruits. Go for variety and a variety of recipes. You'll find yourself eating tastier foods than ever.

Try to eliminate cholesterol-containing foods for at least one week. If you can do this, your taste buds will be purified, and you'll find your fruits, vegetables, and grains even more tasty. You might even decide to eliminate cholesterol-containing foods for good.

Watch out for sugared cereals. When possible, make your own cereals from whole grains like couscous, oats, and cornmeal. Barring that, read the labels carefully.

Read the labels even on so-called lite and natural products. A lot of debate lately has focused on just what these labels mean. Several governmental agencies are trying to standardize labeling on foods so they won't be misleading. But thus far, it's "let the buyer beware!"

41

DON'T BELIEVE FOOD LABEL FABLES

AHA Recommendations   The American Heart Association suggests that when shopping we

- read labels carefully,
- check serving sizes,
- count calories and evaluate nutrition content, and
- compare cost per serving and nutrient in each serving.

The Rest of the Story   If we are going to prevent heart disease, we need to know more about reading labels because a lot of the labels are deceptive. Here are some examples of what you'll find on labels that may be deceptive:

- No cholesterol: All this means is the food comes from a plant source. It may be very high in fat and bad for your heart, cholesterol or no. Margarine, for example, is no cholesterol but 100 percent fat.

- Low fat: There is no standard for what low fat means on labeling. A low-fat Italian dressing can be as high as 83 percent fat.
- The percentage of fat: Many labels report percentage fat by weight. Remember that 2 percent milk is really 35 percent fat by calories. Use your Fat Finder's Formula.
- Prime grade beef: Remember that the higher the grade, the higher the fat content. If you must buy beef, you're better off to buy the lower grades because this doesn't mean the quality is inferior, just that there's less fat.
- Lite: Again, there is no standard for what "lite" means. It means anything the manufacturer wants it to.

The NLEA   Fortunately, a new law that will tighten up the labeling and advertising laws, the Nutritional Labeling and Education Act, is supposed to go into force sometime in 1994. This bill will force all manufacturers to state, clearly and concisely, what is really in their foods. This bill will include fresh produce, and there is increasing pressure on the U.S. Department of Agriculture, which regulates meat and poultry, to adopt a similar policy.

Some companies are already beginning voluntary compliance with the new law. Others are ducking and dodging and double-talking themselves to death, trying to keep up the old subterfuge. In the meantime, if you're going to shop wisely and buy what's good for you, you'd better be on your toes. And if you've so far been naive, stop believing food labels!

42

BE A
SMART
COOK

Be a Healthy Chef   I've always believed that good health starts in the kitchen. My onetime professor Dr. William Castilli, a leading expert in cholesterol and heart disease, once said the best way to prevent heart disease is to learn ten good recipes that you like and use them over and over.

Don't Pour Grease Down Your Throat   The first thing you need to learn about food preparation is that you must quit pouring grease down your and your family's throats. We're talking a lot about cholesterol and fats, but this is one lesson you need to learn. The kitchen is another danger area when it comes to the fat-laden SAD.

We drown our taste buds in salt, grease, and sugar. We live on fried foods. They're available everywhere: french fries, fried hamburgers, fried bacon and eggs, fried fillet of fish, fried chicken, fried onion rings. All this grease is collectively being poured down our throats and clogging up our blood vessels—and setting us up for heart disease! When we're cooking at home, fried foods are some of the easiest to prepare. It's time to find alternatives.

Clean Kitchens = Clean Bodies   Did you ever see the kitchen sink of someone who eats a high-fat diet compared to that of someone who does not? Fat is the main reason we need soap to clean our dishes. A strict vegetarian doesn't even need soap to clean dishes because rinsing the dishes with hot water is usually adequate after a fat-free meal. But grease and fats and oils are not water soluble; therefore, they stick to your plates unless you use soap to emulsify them so the water can wash them down the sink. Then the fats clog the "arteries" of your house, just as they clog your own arteries.

Here are a few ideas to get you started on cooking as wisely as possible:

Slow down on the salad dressings   If you sit down to a healthy salad but slather it with fat-based salad dressing, you're kidding yourself. Just about all salad dressings are between 80 and 90 percent fat.

Slow down on the cheese and cream sauces   These sauces are high in cholesterol and fat. Cheddar cheese, for example, is 74 percent fat, and most of it is saturated.

Get rid of your fats, butter, oils, and mayonnaise You'll find it easier to eliminate fats from your diet if they're not even in your kitchen. You can find alternatives that will soon be just as tasty. You can use fat-free dressings and sauces, mustard, fresh lemon or lime juice, or light spices to flavor your foods.

Keep healthy snacks on hand Try eating fresh fruits, vegetable sticks, and air-popped popcorn. Snacking is good for you if you do it right.

These are just a few of the ways you can turn your kitchen into the center for your health. Many good cookbooks can teach you more. Or you can be inventive and come up with some brand-new ideas on your own.

43

EAT SMART WHEN YOU EAT OUT

Behind the Times? Unfortunately, most restaurants are far, far behind the times when it comes to good nutrition. Even most vegetarian restaurants cook with heavy oils and high fat (cheeses) as if they have to make up for the lack of meat by overloading your taste buds.

When You Can't Go Gourmet Still, times are changing. It's not impossible to find a gourmet restaurant or two specializing in low-fat healthy foods in almost every city. Some of them, such as Charlie Trotter's in Chicago and the Greens in San Francisco, have turned whole grain and vegetable dishes into works of art that rival the creations of the world's best chefs. And most cities and even smaller towns offer a variety of ethnic fare, which broadens your possibilities of finding food that is both healthy and tasty. However, many ethnic restaurants have been

Americanized to the point of loading their foods with fat.

What to Look For   Unless you have access to top-notch restaurants that offer healthy fare, you're going to have to make do at an ordinary restaurant. The menu will include meat- or fish-centered entrees with tiny, seldom fresh, vegetable side dishes. Once in a while you even find a vegetarian entree, but it's usually laden with fat. One way to get past this is to forget the entree altogether. Patch a meal together from the side dishes. The salads should be fresh. Select one or two, and hold the dressing. Bring your own oil-free or fat-free dressing if you wish. Then order one or maybe two side dishes of vegetables. A baked potato is usually a good bet if you have the self-control to forget the butter and sour cream. You can salt and pepper it, or otherwise dress it with something low fat, such as steak sauce. Sometimes you're even lucky enough to find steamed veggies on the menu. And then there is the bread, sometimes whole grain. Skip the butter or margarine.

Japanese food, if it's authentically Japanese, offers healthy soups, noodles, vegetables, and other fat-free and tasty dishes. (Stay away from the tempura.) Other ethnic restaurants—Mexican, Middle Eastern, Chinese, Thai—are found in more and more locations and generally offer some healthy and unusual alternatives to salads and side dishes.

Smart Choices Are the Solution   Always remember that most of the entrees on the menu are going to be high in fat and cholesterol. However, that doesn't mean you have to abstain. Just be aware. Center your diet on starchy foods and vegetables. If you must have cholesterol-containing foods and you're celebrating a special occasion, be aware of what you're doing and be sure your meal is as low in fat as possible.

In short, you can indulge yourself occasionally. But if you eat out all the time and you're used to fast foods or other unhealthy fare, you're going to have to make some smart choices if you want to do everything you can to prevent heart disease. There's no other way.

THE
EXERCISE
CONNECTION

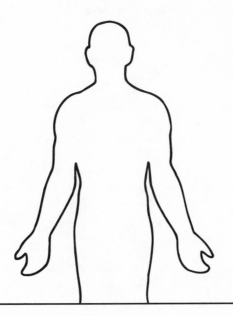

44

UNDERSTAND EXERCISE

A Healthy Heart According to the American Heart Association, getting regular exercise helps prevent heart disease in several ways:

- It improves blood circulation throughout the body. The lungs, heart, and other organs and muscles work together more effectively.
- It improves your body's ability to use oxygen and provide the energy needed for physical activity.
- It helps people handle stress, so they can do more and not tire as easily. It bolsters enthusiasm and optimism.
- It's good for psychological well-being, because it releases tension and helps relaxation and sleep.
- Along with proper diet, it can help people control their weight.[1]

Understand Aerobics At the Aerobics Center in Dallas, Texas, Dr. Kenneth Cooper, the father of aerobics, and his team of experts study the relationship between aerobic exercise, health, and disease. And Dr. Cooper says that aerobic exercise *provides significant protection from heart disease.*

Regular, dynamic aerobic exercise increases the efficiency of the oxygen intake of your body. That means it increases the efficiency of your blood supply and enhances the process of nourishing your various cells. The blood pumps nutrients and oxygen and other wonderful things into these tiny building blocks of life. And no matter how many health-giving nutrients you put into your stomach, it's all for nothing if they aren't properly utilized.

Aerobic exercise helps you by

- tending to increase the level of HDLs in the blood, thereby helping bring your cholesterol into a positive balance.
- increasing your lung capacity, which means longer life span.[2]

But both the AHA and Dr. Cooper are careful to let you know that you should never begin a serious exercise program unless you've first had a checkup and have the okay of your physician. That's especially true if you're older and haven't been exercising for a while or if you already have a serious degenerative illness. Sudden and extreme exercise can stress out an already ailing heart muscle and might even be the catalyst to cause a heart attack. Moderation is the rule of thumb, at least while you're starting out. But if you're in reasonably good health, the following exercises will get you started down the road to total cardiovascular health.

45

TAKE A WALK

Learning to Walk   The simple act of walking can help protect you against heart disease and help save your life. Believe it. Despite the inventions that indulge us and encourage us to be sedentary, walking is one of the best things you can do for yourself.

You can, of course, wear your regular shoes and go for a stroll around the neighborhood every now and again. Or you can turn your walking into a full-on sport, complete with special shoes, gear, specific times of day, and other routines that will help you structure your walking into a serious activity. But if you decide to do this, bear these points in mind:

• Remember to see your doctor before beginning a vigorous walking program. We can't say it too often. People die from sudden and extreme exercise after having been sedentary. These deaths are all too often caused by heart attacks.

- Buy yourself a decent professional pair of walking shoes. A mile or so into your program, you'll be glad you did.
- Invest in other clothing that will make your walks pleasant and comfortable, for instance, a lightweight jacket that will keep you warm if the wind comes up or a pair of loose-fitting slacks or shorts.
- Plan to walk thirty to sixty minutes at least every other day. Start slow, though, perhaps fifteen minutes a day for a week or so, then gradually build up.
- Vary your walking route for maximum pleasure.
- Don't forget to warm up and cool down. Informative books on walking are available at most bookstores. One of them will teach you how.

46

GO
FOR A
SWIM

A Wonderful Exercise   Another treat for your heart is swimming. The American Heart Association tells us that swimming conditions the heart and lungs if performed at the proper intensity for twenty to thirty minutes at a time. If you don't already know how you're missing out on a wonderful exercise. Take the time, and make the effort to learn. But if you do swim and can find a place to indulge yourself, you'll be able to engage in a pleasurable form of aerobic exercise.

One advantage of swimming as an exercise is that it eliminates the strain on joints and bones that can occur from prolonged walking. People who have arthritis or other joint problems can swim to their hearts' content. The ideal schedule for maximum aerobic toning and conditioning is twenty to thirty minutes at least several times a week.

Make the Most of Your Swim

- Check out your local YMCA or YWCA. It offers swimming programs for all ages: underwater exercise programs for seniors, advanced swimming classes for children and teens, and nearly every water sport you can think of.
- If you swim alone but in a safe place, buy a water-resistant Walkman so you can listen to music. It's great fun to practice water ballet on your own.
- Marry your swimming program to another form of exercise, for instance, to walking. Go for a refreshing swim after a long, satisfying walk.
- Take lessons. No matter how well you swim, you can doubtless improve. New strokes and new ways to use your body will make you feel a sense of achievement that can only enhance the new you developing as you proceed with your exercise program. But remember, as with any exercise, if you have a health problem or have been inactive for a long time, check with your physician first.

47

TRY
DANCING

Go for the Full Fitness Package   The American Heart Association tells us that we can improve
our overall health—heart included—by doing aerobic
dancing. This type of dancing can increase available
oxygen, thereby enabling your heart to use oxygen
more efficiently. The AHA is careful to point out,
however, that aerobic dancing or any other form of
exercise cannot help if you insist on ignoring other
major risk factors such as poor diet and smoking.
Any form of exercise, dancing included, must be only
one part of a much larger fitness package if you're
serious about protecting your heart.

But if you are doing everything else you can to
help prevent heart disease, aerobic dancing may be
one welcome addition to the program. And getting
started is easy. You can begin by purchasing one
of the many aerobics videotapes available (Jane

Fonda's are excellent, or perhaps you'll prefer Richard Simmons' "party" for people who love oldies).

Social Dancing   You can join an aerobic dance class—many are open to both men and women, which means you can take your spouse or perhaps meet one there—or you can start your own class! You get a dancing workout while you have the social pleasures of doing your dancing with other people who share your love of health and fitness.

However you decide to dance, these pointers might help you get maximum pleasure from your new activity:

- Invest in some special clothing and/or gear. It will make *you* feel special.
- Join a nonaerobic dance class. Most communities offer ballet classes for all age groups and all degrees of excellence. You can probably find jazz and other modern dance classes, too. Even if you don't plan to aim for the Bolshoi or Broadway, dancing can be fun and can give you a deep sense of accomplishment.
- Design your dancing so you can work out to your favorite type of music. Aerobics tapes run the gamut from spiritual to hard rock. Choosing your favorite will maximize your pleasure.
- Take it seriously. Even when you're alone, working out to a tape, give it your best. You'll get a better workout, and you'll also feel better about yourself.
- Don't forget to warm up and cool down. Most videotapes and audiotapes work these elements into the program. But if you're working out on your own, remember that these two parts of the

workout are vital to keeping your body in top shape.

Again, if you have any real or potential health problems, consult your physician before starting your program.

48

TAKE UP A GROUP SPORT

Do It Your Way   Some of us prefer our own company, and that's okay. Some of us will be perfectly content with a long early-morning bicycle ride in the country, a solitary run, or any of the many other activities that we can do alone.

How to Begin   The possibilities are endless when it comes to innovative ways to indulge in group sports and exercise, no matter what shape you're in. (However, if you have any health problems or if it's been a long time since you've been physically active, please get a physical first, and follow your doctor's advice as you begin your program.)

Group sports and/or exercises come in all levels of expertise. Even if you haven't indulged in a group sport since you were a schoolkid, with a little shopping you can find a group activity that's just right for you. All but the most strenuous of them can be tailored to your physical needs.

- Baseball
- Basketball
- Aerobic dancing
- Bowling
- Tennis
- Golf
- Rowing
- Swimming
- Team running
- Jogging with a friend
- Team bicycling
- Handball or racquetball
- Joining a gym
- Martial arts

Choose One or More   So sit down and do some serious considering. Did you love baseball when you were a youth, but now that you're in your seventies, you don't think you could still hack it? Guess what? There's probably a seniors game somewhere nearby where you could show off your skills. Or maybe you're in your early twenties, but you've just moved to a community and don't know anyone to work out with. Pick up the phone book, then pick up the phone. You'll find community centers or church centers (yes, some churches now have their own gyms) or other centers of activity where you can meet others and share the joy of getting your body into maximum shape so that you and your newfound friends can all look forward to a long and heart-healthy life.

THE
SOCIAL
CONNECTION

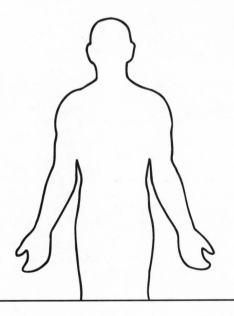

49

LEARN TO BE A TYPE B

Type A People and Heart Disease   Most medical scientists have long suspected that there is more to human health than just well-oiled, well-working machinery. Many suggest that psychological and, yes, spiritual links influence human health.

Drs. Meyer Friedman and Ray Rosenman believed in a link between the psychological, the spiritual, and heart disease way back in the 1950s. They defined a type of behavior they believed was associated with higher risk of heart disease, named the behavior Type A, and began to do research to back up their hypothesis.

They said,

Type A Behavior Pattern is an action complex that can be observed in any person who is aggressively involved in a chronic incessant struggle to achieve more and more in less and less time. . . . Persons possessing this pattern also are quite prone to exhibit free floating but extraordinarily rationalized hostility.[1]

In other words, the Type A person is hostile, self-involved, impatient, and obsessive about interests and goals.

Some Interesting Information   A lot of interesting information came out of Friedman and Rosenman's hypothesis and the subsequent research. But after millions of written words and dozens of research projects, some of the Type A traits that correlated with heart disease appeared to be valid, while others didn't bear up under scientific scrutiny.

Research conducted by Dr. Larry Scherwitz at the University of California, San Francisco, Dr. Redford Williams at Duke University, and others indicates that the parts of Type A behavior that correlate with heart disease are self-involvement, hostility, and cynicism.[2]

To Be or Not to B   Out of the Type A research came another hypothesis: about a Type B personality. This person has all the traits that protect against heart disease. Type B people are nonanxious; they have no time-urgency suffering, no free-floating hostility. They are secure and autonomous, have or court good social skills, play for fun rather than competition, have a strong ability to forgive others for their weaknesses, are patient, have the ability to listen to others, court and preserve meaningful relationships, and are otherwise well connected to society and life. And, oh yes, these people have strong self-esteem.[3]

Who *wouldn't* want to be a Type B? These are the

people most of us admire and even love. Their quali- ties are all the best ones in humanity.

Unfortunately, Type B is just that, an ideal type. Still, most of us have at least some Type B qualities, and we are all capable of changing our behavior. So try to minimize or eliminate your Type A attributes while you polish and perfect your Type B qualities— and learn a few more. It's worth your while to make the effort so you can have a happier, fuller, and (if you protect your heart) longer life.

50

IS LAUGHTER YOUR BEST MEDICINE?

A Very Good Medicine   In 1964, well-known journalist Norman Cousins fell dramatically ill with a rare and serious disease that degenerates the collagen, or connective tissue, throughout the body. The doctors believed the disease to be irreversible. Cousins checked himself out of the hospital and into a hotel. He played funny movies, read humorous books, and did anything else he could think of to provoke laughter.

He initially intended to put himself into a positive frame of mind. But he quickly learned that laughter was also a direct antidote for the intense pain he'd been feeling: ten minutes of laughter would serve as a painkiller for two hours.

Cousins recovered. He promptly told people about what had happened to him. The *New England Journal of Medicine* published an article written by him, and he went on to publish the best-selling book *Anat-*

omy of an Illness as Perceived by the Patient.[1] The rest is history, for now laughter has become an integral part of many therapy groups for patients with all sorts of degenerative diseases.

Neurochemicals   Scientists have learned that there is a certain chemistry associated with happiness and laughter. The physical link is between chemicals manufactured in the brain (neurochemicals) and the body, possibly the immune system. When scientists finally unlock all the mysteries of these chemicals and the ways in which they interact with the rest of the human body, we'll have come a long way toward finding a cure for many serious diseases.

In the meantime, it's sufficient to know that they exist, and that you can tap into them and set them to work for you by having a good laugh. Even though heart disease isn't an immune system disease, laughter also reduces stress, and many studies link stress with tendencies toward heart disease.

However, while laughter can apparently lessen your risk of contracting some diseases, laughter alone is not enough. We must remember that Norman Cousins ultimately died from a heart attack. So, though laughter may have prolonged his life, he may have needed a better diet and even more exercise if he wanted to prevent a heart attack.

So—laugh a little. But don't forget to change your diet and get the right amount of exercise to help you stay healthier and live longer.

51

KNOW
THE JOB
CONNECTION

Don't Work Your Heart Out In the April 11, 1990, issue of the *Journal of the American Medical Association,* Dr. Peter L. Schnall and friends published a study on the relationship between blood pressure and job strain. Their conclusions?

> Job situations where the level of work demands exceeds the individual's ability to control or deal with those demands creates a challenge that activates the sympathetic nervous system and leads to an elevation of BP [blood pressure] at work. Long-term exposure (over years) to job strain is hypothesized to ultimately result in a sustained elevation of BP that then causes structural change in the cardiovascular system.[1]

This structural change comes in the form of a thickened or enlarged heart, a condition that correlates positively with increased risk of heart disease.

In other words, these researchers may have discovered a mechanism by which job strain correlates to coronary heart disease morbidity.

Know When You're Stressed   According to this research, the work conditions defined as *job strain* are:

- high psychological demands with regard to job performance.
- low levels of perceived control over work-related events.

Both components had to be simultaneously present for their definition of job strain to occur.

You can imagine such a situation (perhaps you're even *in* such a situation): forty or so hours per week undergoing an enormous amount of pressure to perform, while at the same time having no control over the ability to perform. It would be like trying to move forward and backward at the same time. Yet, far too many of us work in those conditions.

Change Your Job, or Change Your Coping Strategies   Some people may be able to change jobs to achieve healthier situations. But what if you aren't one of them? What can you do if you can't change jobs? You can change the ways in which you cope with job stress.

Here are a couple of ways you might do this:

- Identify the things (stressors) causing you the most trouble. Think seriously about ways in which you can change the particular things and your reactions to them.

- Learn to take mini-vacations. Take a good book to work with you, find a private place, and learn to go there for five or so minutes at a time. Tune your work out, and read something as far removed from your work experience as possible. If you've always wanted to go to Spain, Japan, or Timbuktu, find books about those places and read tiny segments at a time. Or if time travel is your thing, pick up a couple of interesting history books or books on archaeology or dinosaurs. Or your mini-vacation may be nothing more than five minutes spent in front of a window, watching the blue sky and birds and thinking about your latest fishing trip. Or you may take a short break and go for a brisk walk. Exercise is a great way to lessen stress.

Now that we've got you started, you'll be amazed at the many inventive ways you can take mini-vacations to break up your work. You can increase your level of perceived control and thereby reduce job stress. And there are many other ways. Take time to discover the ones that work for you.

52

SHARE THIS BOOK WITH A FRIEND

You're Only As Healthy As Your Neighbor
At the Waianae Coast Comprehensive Health Center in Hawaii where I serve as Director of Preventive Medicine, we have a saying: "You're only as healthy as your neighbor." What this means is that when we look out for the health of others, we ultimately look out for our own health because what we do influences others and what they do influences us.

So Have a Heart   By reading this book, you have learned what you need to do to protect yourself and your loved ones against heart disease. But what about other people? Remember, nearly a million people are dying in this country each year from cardiovascular disease, and most of it is preventable. Some of these people are your friends, neighbors, church mates, and others near to you.

Over the past few decades we have made strides

toward reducing this epidemic. The rates of heart disease and stroke have fallen over 20 percent, largely due to the individual efforts of people like yourself who are changing their diets and life-styles. Our eating habits have changed as well, for as a nation we are eating less fat today than we did forty years ago, and we are also eating more whole grains and more beans, fresh fruit, and vegetables.

A few short decades ago, people who said that cardiovascular disease could be caused by diet and lifestyle were scoffed at. Today, the causal relationship is well established. This shows that the efforts of individuals *can* make a difference in the nation as a whole. The more people who adopt a healthy lifestyle and diet, the lower heart disease rates will fall. In addition, as more people adopt healthy diets and life-styles, it will become easier for you to continue a healthy diet and life-style. For instance, already at the supermarket we are seeing more and more low-fat foods, a better quality of produce, more breads made with whole grain, and other major improvements in the foods available to us. And it has become easier to find non-smoking sections in public places. There are numerous other improvements.

So share this book with a friend. As God gives us our daily bread, we should give others our daily wisdom. We are all connected, and when we help others, we are really helping ourselves.

Notes

1

1. U.S. Department of Health and Human Services, Public Health Service, *The Surgeon General's Report on Nutrition and Health* (Washington, D.C.: U.S. Government Printing Office, 1988), p. 4.

2

1. All definitions taken from *Reader's Digest Great Encyclopedic Dictionary* (Pleasantville, N.Y.: Reader's Digest Association, 1967).

4

1. Dean Ornish, M.D., S. Brown, and L. W. Scherwitz, "Can Lifestyle Changes Reverse Coronary Heart Disease?" *Lancet* 336 (1990): 129–133.
2. A. Strom, "Mortality From Circulatory Diseases in Norway 1940–1945," *Lancet* 1 (1951): 126.

5

1. W. B. Kannel, W. P. Castelli, and T. Gordon, "Cholesterol in the Prediction of Atherosclerodic Disease: New Perspectives Based on the Framingham Study," *Ann. Internal Med.* 90 (1979): 85.

6

1. Ibid.
2. Strom, "Mortality from Circulatory Diseases," 126.

9

1. I-Min Lee and Ralph S. Pattenbarger, Jr., "Change in Body Weight and Longevity," *Journal of the American Medical Association,* Oct. 21, 1992.

10

1. C. H. Hennekens et al., "Final Report on the Aspirin Component of the Ongoing Physicians' Health Study," *New England Journal of Medicine* 321 (1989): 129–35.

2. Earl Ubell, "The New Powers of Aspirin," *Parade,* May 12, 1991, pp. 12–13 (includes an interview with Dr. Hennekens).

13

1. Kannel, Castelli, and Gordon, "Cholesterol," 85.

17

1. Walter Willet et al., "Relative and Absolute Excess Risks of Coronary Heart Disease Among Women Who Smoke Cigarettes," *New England Journal of Medicine* 317 (1987): 1303–9.
2. American Heart Association National Center, *Smoking and Heart Disease,* No. 51-035-B(CP) (Dallas: American Heart Association, 1986), p. 5.

18

1. J. E. Fielding and K. J. Phenow, "Health Effects of Involuntary Smoking," *New England Journal of Medicine* 319 (1988): 1452–58.
2. Ibid., pp. 1456–57.

21

1. *Medical World News,* July 1992, p. 35.
2. "Test Case for Passive Smoking," *British Medical Journal* 304 (1992): 1529.
3. Ibid.

22

1. Kannel, Castelli, and Gordon, "Cholesterol," 85.

27

1. NIH Publication No. 92-3248, available through the Cancer Information Service, Cancer Research Center of Hawaii, 1236 Lauhala Street, Honolulu, Hawaii 96813.

28

1. A. S. Whittemore et al., "Diet, Physical Activity, and Colorectal Cancer Among Chinese in North America and China," *JNCI* 82 (1990): 915–26.
2. T. T. Shintani et al., "Obesity and Cardiovascular Risk Intervention Through Ad-libitum Feeding of Traditional Hawaiian Diet," *Am. Journal Clin. Nutr.* 53 (1991): 1647S.

3. Dean Ornish, M.D., S. Brown, and L. W. Scherwitz, "Can Life-style Changes Reverse Coronary Heart Disease?" *Lancet* 336 (1990): 129–33.

30

1. Terry T. Shintani, M.D., M.P.H., "The Eat More, Weigh Less Diet," used by permission.

33

1. H. O. Bang and Jorn Dyerberg, "Plasma, Lipids, and Lipoproteins in Greenlandic West Coast Eskimos," *Acta Med. Scan.* 192 (1972): 85–94.
2. D. Kromhout et al., "The Inverse Relationship Between Fish Consumption and 20 Year Mortality from Coronary Heart Disease," *New England Journal of Medicine* 312 (1985): 1205–9.

34

1. K. Dahl Jorgensen, C. Joner, and K. Hanssen, "Relationship Between Cows' Milk Consumption and Incidence of Insulin Dependent Diabetes Mellitus in Childhood," *Diabetes Care* 14 (1991): 1001–3.

36

1. J. T. Dwyer, "Health Aspects of Vegetarian Diets," *Am. Journal Clin. Nutr.*, 48 (1988): 712–38.

38

1. H. Trowell and D. Burkitt, eds., *Western Diseases: Their Emergence and Prevention* (Cambridge: Harvard University Press, 1981).

44

1. American Heart Association, *"E" Is for Exercise,* p. 1. Write the American Heart Association, 7320 Greenville Avenue, Dallas, Texas 75231.
2. K. Cooper, *Aerobics* (New York: Bantam, 1986).

49

1. Cited in Berton H. Kaplan, "Social Health and the Forgiving Heart, the Type B Story," *Journal of Behavioral Medicine* 15 (1992): 3–12.

2. Dean Ornish, M.D., *Dr. Dean Ornish's Program for Reversing Heart Disease* (New York: Ballantine, 1990), p. 86.
3. Kaplan.

50
1. N. Cousins, *Anatomy of an Illness as Perceived by the Patient* (New York: Bantam, 1981).

51
1. Dr. Peter L. Schnall et al., "The Relationship Between 'Job Strain' Workplace Diastolic Blood Pressure, and Left Ventricular Mass Index," *Journal of the American Medical Association* 263 (1990): 1935.